'*Bringing Relationships into Voice Hearing* is an important book which will enlighten and inspire many mental health practitioners, people who hear voices and family members. There is a good balance between theoretical material for practical use of the Tripartite approach and personal reflections and examples of different ways to use the approach. I think it should be in every mental health service Library and available to all practitioners who work with voice hearers.'

Rufus May, *PhD, consultant clinical psychologist*

'*Bringing Relationships into Voice Hearing* is a tour de force, rich in insight, warmth and compassion. Allison and Lafferty's focus on the dynamic tripartite relationships between voice hearers, their voices and practitioners makes an important contribution to the theory and practice of relational approaches to voice hearing that will make a real difference to people's lives. Drawing on lived experience of voice hearing, in-depth empirical research, and the wisdom produced through practical workshops delivered over many years, this book is an inspiration as well as a guide to effecting positive change for people who are distressed by their voices.'

Angela Woods, *Professor of Medical Humanities and director of the Institute for Medical Humanities, Durham University*

Bringing Relationships into Voice Hearing

This book presents a novel, theoretically informed practical approach to voice hearing, which aims to help readers improve relational harmony, reduce distress related to voice hearing, and improve experiences of supportive approaches.

This book presents a Tripartite Relationship Theory, which conceptualises experiences of voice hearing within voice hearer-voice practitioner (or other supporters) relationships. The first part of this book centres on theoretical aspects of the approach, emphasising voice hearers' internal relational experiences with voices and their relational experiences with practitioners, set against a backdrop of mental healthcare, as a way of understanding voice hearing experiences. Shaped by this theoretical relational framework, the second part of this book provides readers with a practical application of how to support voice hearers to feel safe during times of distress, how to nurture helpful relationships, how to understand voice hearing experiences in relation to their life story, and how to "talk with" and "mark-make" with voices.

This book will be accessible to voice hearers, practitioners, and supporters. It provides a framework for understanding the felt experience of voice hearing and how to influence positive change and better relationships with self and voices.

Rob Allison, PhD, is an academic and mental health nurse. He has many years of experience working with and learning from people distressed by voices. He developed a tripartite relationship-grounded theory to help understand and support voice hearing experiences.

Ruth Lafferty, MSc, is an academic and hears voices. She uses her lived experience, creative practice, and psychotherapy training to inform her teaching work with voice hearers and practitioners.

Bringing Relationships into Voice Hearing

Introducing a Tripartite Relationship Theory

Rob Allison and Ruth Lafferty

Routledge
Taylor & Francis Group
LONDON AND NEW YORK

Designed cover image: "Family Snap" (2024) Ruth Lafferty, water colour on paper.

First published 2025
by Routledge
4 Park Square, Milton Park, Abingdon, Oxon OX14 4RN

and by Routledge
605 Third Avenue, New York, NY 10158

Routledge is an imprint of the Taylor & Francis Group, an informa business

© 2025 Rob Allison and Ruth Lafferty

The right of Rob Allison and Ruth Lafferty be identified as authors of this work has been asserted in accordance with sections 77 and 78 of the Copyright, Designs and Patents Act 1988.

This work was supported by the University of York.

Trademark notice: Product or corporate names may be trademarks or registered trademarks, and are used only for identification and explanation without intent to infringe.

British Library Cataloguing-in-Publication Data
A catalogue record for this book is available from the British Library

ISBN: 978-1-032-61986-6 (hbk)
ISBN: 978-1-032-61984-2 (pbk)
ISBN: 978-1-032-61991-0 (ebk)

DOI: 10.4324/9781032619910

Typeset in Times New Roman
by codeMantra

Contents

Preface

Welcome to our book! We wrote this to share some of our own experiences regarding voice hearing in the hope that it helps readers struggling with difficult voice hearing experiences, including anyone trying to support someone who is struggling. We hope you enjoy reading it and find it to be helpful.

Voice hearing can be frightening and debilitating for all concerned, despite efforts to find numerous and varied ways to cope with the voices. The focus of our work has been on helping people (and their supporters) who have felt distressed by their voices. For several years, we have delivered workshops focussing on voice hearing, attended by practitioners and people distressed by voices, where we have met many generous and inspiring people. We are grateful to them all for sharing their experiences and contributing to our own learning about voice hearing.

We have learnt many things about voice hearing over the past few years, in our training workshops, through reading and through our respective academic work. We have learnt by listening to thoughtful reflections and curious questions from voice hearers, practitioners, and family members. This process of questioning is what expanding knowledge is all about and finding the right questions to ask about voice hearing and listening to the responses of everyone, including voices has become our imperative.

We want to keep sharing knowledge and asking questions. The exercises we suggest in Part 3 are vehicles to explore the individual experience of voice hearing from a voice hearer's perspective so they can ask their own questions related to where they are in their voice hearing experience. The significance of this questioning has pushed forward our own enquiry as these questions represent the edge of people's knowledge and their desire to know more. We have sought to explore these questions in the workshops and these vital discussions drove us to write this book. Answering these questions, however, must be a collective process. No one person, and certainly not us, has all the answers. The moment we think we have a universal answer for other people, we have taken power away from someone who makes sense of their voices in a different way. The only universal principle we have identified is about the primacy of the relationships between voice hearer, voices, and others in the voice hearer's world. Voice hearers, practitioners, and ourselves are all on the same quest of trying to understand the voice hearing experience and ways to help voice hearers have a better life by listening to and responding to voices in a productive relational way.

A key aim of ours throughout these workshops has been to foster shared learning opportunities for all participants, including ourselves, to increase knowledge and understanding of voice hearing experiences. More specifically, we have sought to identify ways to reduce distress associated with voice hearing and increase harmony within voice hearing experiences. We want to transfer our learning from these experiences into this book. We want to reach out through our writing to those who struggle with their voice hearing experiences and to those who want to support people who hear voices. We hope readers can learn more about voice hearing and become more confident and capable of either living with voices or providing support to people who hear voices.

For those readers who do hear voices, you may notice that your voices comment on your reading even at this early stage of the book. You may even experience your voices becoming agitated or increasingly hostile or threatening as you read and make your way through the pages of this book. So, we would like to offer reassurance right from the outset. Through writing this book, we hope that readers who hear voices can work towards a better way of *being with* their voices. We would like to make it clear to your voices that this book is not intended to be of any threat to them. In fact, we believe voices can be a valuable historical link from which voice hearers can make sense of their own personal stories and evolve into their future selves. As such, we believe it is helpful to learn how to value voices in order to better understand them and their role in the lives of voice hearers.

This is not to dismiss the distress and difficulties encountered by many people who hear voices. If you are struggling with your voices, it might seem impossible to consider them as anything but an abusive and unwelcome presence in your life. One of us (Ruth Lafferty (RL)) can relate to this through several years of difficult voice hearing experiences. For RL, exploring ways to create more harmony with and between her voices has been a journey of discovering connections, uncovering missing pieces, and finding allies in voices to grapple with distress. As you read this book, we encourage you to remain open to the possibility that you can improve your voice hearing experiences by changing the relationships with your voices and with yourself, despite having understandable doubts.

Many reasons have been put forward to explain why some people hear voices. Some of these reasons have held more sway than others. Before we get into any detail about voice hearing in the first part of this book, though, we want to be clear from the outset on our position regarding voice hearing. Influenced by our own work and that of others (e.g., Marius Romme, Sandra Escher, Rufus May, Eleanor Longdon, Rachel Waddingham, Ron Coleman, and Angela Woods closely associated with the broader voice hearing community), we advocate for individual sense-making of voice hearing experiences. Aligned with a broadly accepted biopsychosocial perspective, we accept that all our sensory experiences are products of biological processes but, importantly, happen within sociological contexts, and psychologically are uniquely interpreted and experienced. More specifically, we believe that voice hearing experiences are rooted in the life history of the hearer and their related interpretation of these historical roots.

However, we do not believe we or others are sufficiently expert to impose causal explanations that might help individuals understand why they hear voices. Rather, we believe the voice hearers themselves have the potential to become their own experts through investigating their own life history and finding meaning. That is, it is important for individuals to develop their own personal meaning concerning their voice hearing experience. As such, we align with a philosophy in which we believe we all can construct personal meaning and explanation regarding our experiences. For many people, voice hearing can be distressing, frightening, and overwhelming, which can make it difficult to reach an understanding. It is our intention to share our learning in this book to help voice hearers along their own journeys to find personal and meaningful understandings of their own voice hearing. The approaches we share throughout this book are rooted in this worldview.

We recognise there might be potential conflict for some readers regarding the position we take concerning voice hearing while at the same time advocating for individual explanations. How can we favour one particular worldview on voice hearing yet also advocate the importance of developing an individual and potentially different or even contrasting personal worldview? Our answer to this is rooted in the notion of power. This is something we will return to throughout this book but, for now, we think it is important to state that voice hearing is at its core about power. Reclaiming power is an essential part of one's journey towards improved voice hearing experiences. So, as best as we can, we not only try to be transparent but also suspend our perspective on voice hearing to provide space for individuals to develop their own sense of what they experience.

We should also offer another potential conflict at this early point in this book, which concerns the terms we use to describe people, which we recognise may read as labelling and for that we apologise. We use the term "voice hearer". This is a term commonly used by people who hear voices, and we also use it to improve the flow of some of our discussion points. Similarly, regarding our use of the term "patient", we recognise that many people will not have accessed healthcare services and, therefore, will not consider this to be a term relevant to their personal experiences. However, we occasionally use this term as it reflects broader common parlance, a term typically referred to in the wider literature. We also wish to acknowledge that some of the uncensored reports of what voices say include profane terms that may provoke a negative reaction. It is not our intention to cause offence or to use these examples in a gratuitous way. They are relevant to our discussions and the real experience of living with distressing and distressed voices. After deliberation, we thought it essential not to censor voice content as this sanitises the voice hearing experience and would feel irrelevant to voice hearers who struggle with one of the very difficult aspects of the voice hearing experience, which is the emotional impact of regular difficult-to-hear voice content. We wish our work to be relevant, congruent, and honouring of voice hearers who struggle, often silently with this aspect of their experience and the shaming that can occur as a consequence. We deliberately bring this taboo aspect into the light so that voice hearers do not need to feel alone with it and to encourage voice hearers and those who help to make meaning of voice content where it is relevant and look underneath the language to what this raw distress might relate to without attaching too much to the profane language itself. Finally, we also refer to the term voice hearing throughout this book but much of what we discuss may also be useful to readers who struggle with seeing things that others do not and to those who have unusual strong beliefs that can interrupt daily life and provoke equally strong emotions affecting mood, daily functioning, and relationships. Happy reading!

About the designed cover image

Bringing Relationships into Voice Hearing: Introducing a Tripartite Relationship Theory

"Family Snap" (2024) Ruth Lafferty, water colour on paper.

"Family Snap" is an abstract image inspired by the voice mapping exercise described in Chapter 7.

Relationships with my voices evolve in circles and cycles, each impacting the other in a room, in space, around my head, in my sleep. My voices form collectives. If not with me, then amongst themselves. We are always communing somewhere and somehow, in ignorance, in anger, in love, in awe, in spite of my clumsy attempts to connect with them or run away from them and from myself when the nausea bites. My voices are never static. They rush towards or circle calmly, they stand and brace me or fly at my very soul. They heal and wound. Then when I can see and hear, they bring the light and I perceive them wounding no more. They invite me to weave a new way of living with new colours and patterns I've never lived before. They compel me to be brave and, one by one, to embrace them all.

Part 1

Introduction

Some people who hear voices feel untroubled by them or feel sufficiently able to cope with them without the need for further support. Indeed, voice hearing can enrich their lives. In fact, a large minority, for example, 30% in an online survey by Woods, Jones, Alderson-Day, Callard, & Fernyhough (2015) have reported their voices to be positive and helpful. However, for many people, voice hearing can be nonsensical and distressing. Many of you reading this book, especially those who hear voices, will know that voice hearing is an incredibly powerful experience impacting your entire life: your emotions, how you think, the actions you take, and even the physical feelings you might notice in your body. Additionally, for readers who do not hear voices, but who want to support those who do hear voices, you might struggle to understand what voice hearing is and how it is experienced.

Although people can have similar experiences of voice hearing, we are all individuals. No two people have the exact same experience; voice hearing experiences are unique. As such, we have avoided writing a step-by-step guide to resolve *all* the difficulties for *everyone* relating to distressing voices. We believe it is important to encourage and support people who hear voices to develop their own explanation in a way that makes personal sense. Adopting non-meaningful explanations can increase the tension between voice hearers and their voices and contribute towards internal/intrapersonal disharmony. Instead, this book aims to help people establish their own understanding of voice hearing, provide a range of activities that can help make sense of the particularities of their own voices, and provide options that can alleviate at least some of the distress they might cause.

In Part 1 of this book, we provide an overview of voice hearing and conventional approaches taken to support people distressed by it, set against a wider sociopolitical context. In Part 2, we introduce readers to the Tripartite Relationship Theory, which sets out voice hearing in a context of relationships between voice hearers, their voices, and practitioners (or other people). This theory informs Part 3, where we explore a range of activities that have emerged from working with people who hear voices, and we encourage readers to be creative in their application of these to find personal solutions to living with a range of difficult and distressing experiences. In this opening chapter, we first consider how commonly reported voice hearing is before we then explore how it is experienced.

DOI: 10.4324/9781032619910-1

Chapter 1

Introduction

An overview of voice hearing

How common is voice hearing?

Voice hearing can be experienced by anyone and across the lifespan. It is typically associated with emotional distress and, for many people distressed by it, experienced in mental healthcare settings or treatment contexts. Perhaps surprisingly, it has been associated with numerous non-mental health conditions, including endocrine-related metabolic conditions such as thyroid function, chromosomal disorders, autoimmune disorders, acquired immunodeficiency disorders (HIV/AIDS), sleep disorders, neurological events, traumatic brain injuries, cardiovascular events, and neurodegenerative conditions (Waters & Fernyhough, 2017). However, evidence suggests that voice hearing is more commonly associated with conditions such as affective disorder and personality disorder (Choong, Hunter, & Woodruff, 2007) and is mostly investigated in relation to psychosis (Pierre, 2010) and schizophrenia (Larøi, 2012).

Although some people who hear voices will have a diagnosis of a health condition of some sort, some will not. Voice hearing has been reportedly experienced by people termed by researchers as healthy individuals or, in other words, the wider general population (Johns et al., 2014; Larøi et al., 2012; Beavan, Read, & Cartwright, 2011; Sommer et al., 2010). For example, from a survey of 153 people hearing voices, Woods, Jones, Alderson-Day, Callard, and Fernyhough (2015) found that most had a formal diagnosis, schizoaffective disorder being the most common (16%), but a good proportion (18%) had no diagnosis. The prevalence of voice hearing experienced in the general population has been reported as 6% of the population (Linscott & Van Os, 2013), 7.3% (Kråkvik et al., 2015), and 5%–13% (Beavan, Read, & Cartwright, 2011). Interestingly, from a sample of 2,533 respondents to a questionnaire in a Norwegian study regarding voice hearing, those who heard voices but had not sought professional help outnumbered those who had sought help by 140 to 30, approximately 84% (Kråkvik et al., 2015).

A question arising from these findings of voice hearing in the wider "non-clinical" general population is: what is the difference between people who hear voices but are in receipt of healthcare support and people who hear voices but receive no healthcare support? Findings from a range of investigations that have

DOI: 10.4324/9781032619910-2

compared voice hearing in the general population with people with a diagnosis of schizophrenia suggest numerous commonalities regardless of whether the person has a formal diagnosis or not. For example, there might be common experiences of anxiety and depression (Lawrence, Jones, & Cooper, 2010) and a history of trauma (Daalman et al., 2012; Lataster et al., 2006; Romme, Escher, Dillon, Corstens, & Morris, 2009). Key differences between clinical and non-clinical populations, however, include negative content and severity of voices, the harmful impact of this on the voice hearer's functioning, and the older age at which the person hears voices (Larøi, 2012). Returning to the above cited Krakvik study, compared to those who hadn't sought professional help, voice hearers who sought professional help were more likely to experience negative feelings/emotions (anxiety, loneliness, sadness, uncertainty, jealousy, aggression), report daily and negative voices, hear their voices commenting upon them, and more likely to react to commanding voices (including begging their voices to keep silent). Bless et al. (2018) analysed data from the Krakvik study and compared voice hearers who had reported a specific adverse life event at the first onset of their voice hearing with those who had not reported such an event. They concluded that the presence of an adverse life event was associated with more troublesome voices.

So, as we have briefly highlighted, not all voice hearers have a diagnosis of a mental health condition (Beavan, Read, & Cartwright, 2011), and many do not seek or need professional help (Sommer et al., 2010). We believe that such a wide range of diagnostic and non-diagnostic associations with voice hearing limits any meaningful diagnostic value. However, it seems clear that there are important differences between people who are in receipt of healthcare compared to those in the general population regarding voice hearing. We have written this book with the aim of supporting people distressed by voice hearing, regardless of whether a person has been given a diagnosis.

What is voice hearing?

The term voice hearing is an umbrella term for a range of sensory phenomena, including hearing an audible voice(s), having a sense of a specific recognisable presence, a presence dominated by a sensation such as dread, audible sounds that are not verbal but have an emotive quality such as crying or growling, and seeing visions or inanimate objects taking on an animate power. The experience of voices can start with one voice or several at the same time, and they can grow in number or recede over time. The voices may be recognisable from the past or present, unrecognisable or a mixture. They can be deafeningly loud to barely audible and may change depending on where the person is, who they are with, and what is happening around them. They can be perceived as supportive, distressing, distressed, neutral or silent, and often a mixture of these, and they can change over time. We explore this in more detail when we introduce voice mapping in Chapter 7.

Put simply, voice hearing refers to the hearing of a voice or number of voices in the absence of a speaker (Waters, 2010). Starting to hear voices can be a shocking and bewildering experience. They can start suddenly or emerge over time in a way that can be hard to identify. They can start at any age, and the number of voices a person may hear can range from one to hundreds. They may be volatile and hurtful or soothing and supportive, or a mixture. Voices can be of any age, gender, or genderless and have distinct personalities or share some recognisable qualities with the voice hearer or other people who have been a part of the voice hearer's life. They may be invisible to the voice hearer but can be heard from specific places such as behind a wall or in parts of the hearer's body. By contrast, a voice hearer may be able to see them clearly or they may be shadowy, ghost-like, or just out of sight. They may also know what their voices look like without seeing them in the room. Voices can present in a myriad of ways that are as individual as a fingerprint.

In addition to being personal to the hearer, voices can also change over time. They can also remain unchanged in time and space; for example, a voice may always remain eight years old, or the voice may age with the voice hearer. Voices can disappear for long periods of time and return months or years later, often at a significant point or stressful experience in the voice hearer's life. The effect they can have on day-to-day life and the sense a person might make of themselves can be devastating and make it very hard for them to relate to this disturbing new world. This is often due in part to the shock of starting to hear and experience something that others do not and the oppressive language or communications that distressing voices typically use. Voices that are distressing usually use language that can be profane, accusatory, derogatory, and instructive to harm self or others, and voices also seem to have an uncanny knack of speaking about the voice hearer in the most personally hurtful way. What may distress one voice hearer may not distress another. It is the tailor-made quality that can be so distressing and irksome in a voices' ability to be so specific to the voice hearer's deepest hurts. Alongside distressing voice content, a voice hearer may also experience physical sensations such as nausea, headaches, bodily pain, and sensations such as being hit, rained on or being touched. One of us (Ruth Lafferty (RL)) had very regular nausea in the first couple of years of hearing voices and can feel a sharp shove in the back connected to certain commands from a specific voice. A certain smell can also accompany a voice or type of communication. In addition to seeing voices or images, a voice hearer can experience blurred vision or sensations through other senses, which can add to the intensity of the voice hearing experience. Strong complex and debilitating emotions associated with the content of a voice increases the difficulty for the voice hearer to manage themself, their voices and their daily tasks and relationships with others.

Not only can a person who hears voices encounter difficult and distressing experiences with a voice (or numerous voices), but this can also extend to other people. The following two quotes from research by one of us (RA) illustrate the difficulty not just for the person hearing voices but for others too (we explore this research in more detail in part two):

> My own kind of anxious avoidant pattern of relating is manifested in the way that I've learned to relate to the voices.
>
> (Bella, voice hearer)

…if someone is very, very distressed by voices, it's kind of heart-breaking, isn't it? You want to intervene. It seems cruel not to do something…[but]… I suppose you're damned if you do it and damned if you don't do it. Sometimes it feels like you're stuck between a rock and a hard place.

(Carrie, practitioner)

Extending the above quotations, we believe that voice hearing is about relationships. From the above two quotes, we can see that voice hearing can affect not only the person hearing voices but also their relationships with other people and for other people, too, who might try to offer support. It concerns the ways in which a person hears their voices and, consequently, their intra-personal (or internal) relating with their voices; and it concerns the ways in which they inter-personally (or externally) interact with other people who might try to offer support. As such, we believe voice hearing is about relating, both with voices and other people. Later in part two, we introduce readers to a tripartite "voice hearer-voice practitioner" relationship as a theoretical explanation of voice hearing experiences.

In her statement above, Bella crystallises a major dilemma for many voice hearers with distressing voices, and that is how to relate to voices in a disconnected way to maintain a stable path in day-to-day life. It can be lonely trying to navigate new experiences especially, as is common, if you are trying to keep the experience to yourself for fear of voices carrying out threats if you talk about them, or fear that others might change their view of you, or fear of being hospitalised and diagnosed with a mental disorder. Equally, this may be welcome when desperate for an explanation. But so often, at the very point when a person needs compassionate understanding and support, it may be the very time they feel they cannot reach out for fear of making their life worse, even if they felt there was someone in their life they could trust enough to talk with about their experiences. This cycle of escalating distress and silencing oneself can result in isolation from the rest of one's social world and risks developing a sense of being forever different to others. It may also be reinforced by distressed and suspicious sounding voices that often encourage a voice hearer to not trust and not speak. This is a specific and very real challenge for many voice hearers. We encourage readers to find a self-compassionate way of supporting oneself if this is a recognisable cycle of isolation and a wish to find more rewarding ways to connect with self, voices, and others. This way of relating is something we will explore in more detail in Part 3.

Hearing voices and responding to their content also lead voice hearers to make changes to their behaviour in different ways. Significantly, voices are experienced as "other". They say things and may encourage the hearer to do things that do not chime with the kind of person they perceive themselves to be. Many voice hearers can feel immense pressure from the voices that excessively comment or advise or even coerce the hearer to engage in certain behaviours. For example, the voice hearer may be more careful about whom they meet and the places they go, not wanting to be too far from where they live. Voices may be instructive about the kind of food a hearer eats and, consequently, a voice hearer might change their diet and consequently eat in a way that is not in accordance with what they would normally choose. People who hear voices make choices every day about all sorts of things, and their voices can heavily influence their decisions if they are not mindful of their own self-agency. It can feel like being micro-managed and, whilst some of the advice may be beneficial, unless a voice hearer feels in charge of the decision, autonomy is compromised and can neutralise the benefits of a good choice. For example, a voice hearer may hear a voice using derogatory terms if they smoke a cigarette. Whilst the voice may have a healthy reason for deterring a voice hearer from smoking, the oppressive energy can make a voice hearer resistant to the good part of the warning and just hear the message as a put-down. This is an area that can be complex for voice hearers, and we believe that forming a more equal relationship with voices that includes negotiation and reasoning can help people to empower their day-to-day decision-making and relieve some of the pressure from what can be perceived as controlling and disempowering voice hearing experiences.

These challenges can have an impact on physical energy. Tiredness and diffi-culty concentrating can make simple tasks difficult and complicated tasks almost impossible when voices are very intense. This is important for voice hearers to acknowledge and give themselves permission for self-care. Allowing time to recharge energy can be a challenge in itself and is something we will return to in Part 3. During the initial period of voice hearing, being able to find some space to make sense of one's voices in a way that feels personal to the voice hearer can be a vital step towards managing and navigating this very difficult and often disturbing phase. Profiling and mapping voices and communicating with voices, which we discuss in later chapters, can help individuals construct personal meaning regard-ing voices generally, including meaning associated with what they say.

The first time of hearing voices can feel like living in a horror story, tailor-made to the person with all the most excruciating aspects of their lived experienced on constant repeat. To voice hearers, it can sound like spinning a futile and negative narrative that is impossible to escape from. It is not impossible but requires empathy, compassion, and a reminder to the voice hearer to be self-caring and patient with themselves and their voices whilst they find their specific keys to unlock the matrix that traps them. Because of the varied and personal nature of voice hearing, it is hard for voice hearers, practitioners, and supporters to find literature or "techniques" to speak into the voice hearer's very specific experience. Our hope is that through this book, we can support voice hearers to find a way that is as specific as their voice hear-ing experience, through profiling, mapping voices, talking with voices, mark-making, and any combination of these that fits the needs and aspirations of the voice hearer.

Sometimes, a voice hearer might struggle to respond when commanded by a voice to do something, especially if it concerns harming oneself or others. Voices can often make threats to a voice hearer if they fail to obey commands, which can create a double-bind. One of RL's voices would tell her that he would harm her family if she went out of the home. The thought of risk of family members being harmed because of a voice hearer's actions (i.e., going out of her house) creates a trap and a reduction in self-agency if she obeys the voice's command or guilt and fear for her family's safety if she disobeys the voice.

How do people describe their voice hearing?

A small proportion of people report to hear a single voice, but most people experience more than one (Woods, Jones, Alderson-Day, Callard, & Fernyhough, 2015). In a recent survey (Brewin et al., 2022), respondents reportedly heard an average of four separate, and mostly male, voices. Furthermore, some people report their voices to include a collection such as crowds, gangs, or groups (Woods, Jones, Alderson-Day, Callard, & Fernyhough, 2015). Sometimes, the hearing of voices is distinct from one's own voice, but it might also be indistinguishable from one's own thoughts. In an interesting analysis of voice hearer's accounts, Wilkinson and Krueger (2022) critique transcriptions from interviews with people describing their voices. They refer to a paradox of voice hearing wherein voice hearing can be "described as being both like and unlike voices heard in everyday life (often simultaneously)" (p. 131). Although we use the term "voices", it is not true to say that all voice hearers hear "voice" content. A small proportion of respondents (9%) from a survey by Woods, Jones, Alderson-Day, Callard, and Fernyhough (2015) reportedly experienced thought-like voices, i.e., they compared their voices to how they experience thoughts. Most of the respondents still described these as voices. A larger proportion (44%) reported their experiences to be indistinguishable from other voices or sounds, i.e., similar to the sound of voices or sounds in the room, and more than a third (37%) reportedly experienced a mix of the two (Woods, Jones, Alderson-Day, Callard, & Fernyhough, 2015).

For many people, voice hearing can be all consuming and disempowering. Voice hearers report a range of emotions associated with their voices, but mostly experience fear and anxiety, and most people report changes in bodily experience when they hear voices (Woods, Jones, Alderson-Day, Callard, & Fernyhough, 2015). Interestingly, Woods and colleagues found that a relatively small proportion of people (14%) reportedly experience shame. Although voices are personal to the hearer in that only they can hear and experience them, voice hearing is more than this. For some, a symbolic identity, informed by interpersonal, political, and cultural contexts, is attributed to voice hearing (Woods, 2013). In other words, the experience of voice hearing can shape the way in which a person perceives themselves and how they predict others perceive them.

Voice content can sometimes help the voice hearer to identify who the voices might be (Brewin et al., 2022; Birchwood & Chadwick, 1997), the extent to which varies across different studies. Woods and colleagues (2015) found that people mostly described their voices as person-like entities with distinct characteristics (age, gender, patterned emotional responses, and intentions). Voices can also take on many forms but, for many people, can be identifiable by the voice hearer as specific people, can vary in age and gender, and sometimes can involve a religious tone, i.e., the Devil or God. For example, Woods and colleagues (2015) found that 22% of respondents to their study reported they recognised their voices as specific, existing individuals; 16% described their voices as supernatural or spiritual entities. People also tend to describe their voices in either positive or negative terms

(Beavan, 2013), although recent research (Brewin et al., 2022) suggests this is mostly negative and a mix of negative and positive, and where voices perceived as belonging to young children to have less negative content compared to voices belonging to adolescents or older age groups.

Voice hearing can also be accompanied by other sensory experiences such as smell, visual presence, taste, or even a feeling across certain parts of the body. These sensations can add to the assault on the senses. Some people might not "hear" their voice at all but can sense their presence; some might hear their voice(s) communicate in a way they can't understand, such as a noise of some sort or an unrecognisable language. We have worked with a person who heard one of their voices as a young baby who could only cry (rather than talk). Some people hear their voices from inside their head, but others can hear them from a range of locations outside of their head (Beavan, 2013). This seems to be a more important distinction for some practitioners than people hearing voices, though, which relates historically to a clinical judgement that voices heard from inside the head are "pseudo" voices. Interestingly, half of respondents to a study by Woods et al. (2015) reported their voices as internally located, with the other half reporting theirs to be externally located.

Some voices can speak in a way that can erode self-confidence, dignity, privacy, and self-worth. Often, because of the threats voices can make, even if they are spoken about to another person, it may be a very long time before a voice hearer speaks about their voices. Equally, it can stir a dread of being seen as quintessentially "mad", fearing what others will make of them or fearing that a process of being pathologised, medicated, and hospitalised will commence and life will spin out of control even further. It is often a very delicate pathway in finding a way to speak about voices and visions for fear of making one's own internal world much more distressing. A primary factor that can affect a voice hearer's courage to talk about their voice hearing is whether there is someone in their life whom they trust enough to tell and whether they can trust themselves to tolerate the uncertainties of speaking about the invisible world in which they live with sufficient confidence that the voice can't enact any threat. Equally, a voice hearer may be desperate to talk about their voices in the hope of getting some kind of help or explanation for the experience.

In Chapter 3, you will meet a number of generous voice hearers who took part in the research for the Tripartite Relationship Theory. They all reported keeping their voice hearing experience private for varied amounts of time. Most feared not being believed; Bella feared being perceived as delusional and Edith also feared receiving a diagnosis of schizophrenia. Many voice hearers hear their voices command them not to trust others and are anxious that the inevitable backlash from their voices for speaking about their voices will make their voices even more difficult to cope with. Practitioners can positively contribute to a voice hearer's experience of first disclosing voices by simply believing them and reassuring them by acknowledging the voices are an important part of the voice hearer's life and by giving them space to explore voices and being respectfully curious about them. This is important to know for anyone supporting a voice hearer. The personal nature of voice hearing makes the experience of hearing voices dynamic and complex. We return to this later in this book in Chapters 6–8.

Box 1.1   RLs' experience of voice hearing

Although hearing a voice(s) is different and personal for each person who hears them, there may be something from my experience that many voice hearers may be able to identify, and so I share it here.

I believe voice hearing is not a clinical experience of a mental illness. Voices speak the stories of our lives and bid us to come closer to all the chapters in it in order to own, honour and embrace the wholeness of our life stories. This includes distress, damage, triumphs, conflicts, and all.

The voices I hear and see started to emerge approximately 14 years ago (at the time of writing) over a period of about two years. I experienced the first voice as an invisible angry entity who suddenly started screaming furious insults in my left ear. Who, or what, was that? Two days later I heard similar words again. This time I heard the words moving about in the space around me. A male voice. The disembodied words were insulting me: "Stupid"; "You useless bastard"; "You fucking stupid ..."; "You brainless ...", words I don't want to write. The words ridiculed what I looked like, how I moved, and what I was. There was jeering derision when I dropped a book I was holding. My first observation was that these critical words came from this entity and was responding to what I was doing. They weren't just random words but targeted at and relating to me. These first few days were wildly destabilising. Was I hearing a ghost? I don't believe in ghosts. Was it someone playing tricks? Was I lucid dreaming? Was there a foggy outline where the voice emanated from? Was I making this up by imagining something to make sense of this outrageous experience? It could have been just my imagination because I had already started experiencing anxiety along with nightmares, intrusive thoughts, and memories about something that had happened many years before. More mocking laughter. Was that the same voice? Now there seemed to be two voices. One mocking, one angry. Voice One was angry. Voice Two laughed hysterically and sneered at things I tried to say back to him. I felt scared by Voice One and humiliated and ashamed when Voice Two burst into the air around me. In my mind's eye, I could see him covering his mouth and pointing at how ridiculous I was to him.

Then three or possibly four more started shrieking, laughing, shouting obscenities in what seemed like unison. One voice first appeared as an 11-foot-high man that I recognised from long-ago. This terrified me to the point of vomiting and freezing when near too many people I didn't know. He would scream instructions, threatening to kill me in many different ways. Another one would "slap" me and snarl that he would kill me if I obeyed the other voices' instruction. A young child's voice emerged and would follow me everywhere, sobbing. Should I try to help this sobbing sound? but it all scared me too much to turn round to this young child, who wasn't there and whom I didn't believe in.

Different voices repeated descriptions of previous distressing experiences on a loop, and the more I ran or tried to distract myself, the more they seemed to follow and find new ways to entrap and humiliate me. I hated myself and the voices that had parachuted into my world one after another. My senses had been possessed by unbidden and unwelcome monstrous ghosts. I became vigilant and strained to hear these foreign things in an attempt to locate where, identify who, predict when, and work out the interminable why. Why were these voices and words coming at me? I started to experience exhaustion, panic, more exhaustion, self-disgust, and all the time voices became more intense and finally became constant. There was no space between the mash-up of conflicted words, images, and sensations. They were already whispering or shouting when I awoke and were still tutting and muttering their disappointment when I went to sleep. I needed to tell someone, a psychiatrist, but didn't want a terminal diagnosis. But I had family and an employer that I needed to answer to, and as much as I was trying to contain this growing "insanity" and minimise the outward signs of shaking and appearing odd, I was failing to manage.

This emergent experience was confusing and difficult to own and describe to others and very difficult for others to understand and tolerate. I felt nauseous regularly and started making myself sick to get rid of the nausea and hoping to vomit away the voices. I felt like I'd entered a different world where the rules had changed and I could not trust what I saw, heard, felt, or touched. I ranged between panic and trying to gather myself into something presentable to my family, friends and kind colleagues who visited me. I was aware that I was responding to voices that others couldn't hear or see. I felt humiliated that I was being perceived as mad and unstable and so focused on trying to remain as "normal" as possible to others.

The cost of this was to use non-prescription drugs and unhelpful patterns of behaviour to attempt to achieve this socially acceptable self in an attempt to avoid fragmenting entirely and to stay as responsible to others as possible. I was trying to make sense of this new reality whilst being aware that something dramatic had changed for others too. Trying to make sense of my internal experience was as much driven by a need to appear sufficiently ok to others to protect them whilst at the same time trying to find ways to ask for help and trying to understand and manage the experience alone.

I tried many things to help me cope including running, long walks often up mountains, restricting my diet to manage nausea, and various prescription drugs that repeatedly failed to eliminate or calm voices. Whilst there were days when I could maintain some kind of external control by trying to be kind and helpful to others, I know I was also increasingly unbearable to be around. Fear of the meaning of these voices and my frustration with myself for not being able to manage them or explain myself leaked out in anger. Increasingly, I was harming myself to try and assuage the level of aggression from the most dominant voices, and I finally felt like I couldn't spin any more plates. Killing myself seemed a plausible option, and engaging in a serious suicide plan that I had been brewing for several months shocked me into submitting to an assessment, and I was hospitalised. I wanted to die, but I couldn't hurt my dearest friends, beautiful nieces, nephews, brother, and sister.

In the end, I found that relationships are the most powerful dynamic and strongest driver. And so, a better way forward began. Not because of anything constructive I experienced in an overcrowded and under-staffed hospital ward, although those weeks were formative in the way I started to view how the world and psychiatry viewed voice hearing. I witnessed people stuck in their voice hearing nightmares with no one to talk to about it, except one compassionate support worker. Because I could see and hear what my fellow voice hearers wanted and needed, I could identify it in myself. They wanted to talk about their experience, reduce their medications so they could think about what they were experiencing, be accepted and understood. Several of my peers on the ward talked about their life experiences and were convinced that these life events were directly related to their voice hearing experience. These conversations and observations chimed with my own beliefs about the intrinsic connections between life experiences and "symptoms".

When I was able to negotiate a subversive discharge from hospital, I wanted to take charge of my own path. I wanted to change the relationship I had with my voices. I couldn't articulate that at the time, but I was using my own self-agency to give up medication and to start on a journey of meaning-making that made sense to me in terms of the way I saw human functioning and distress. I wanted change and to find the guts to stop running and face what looked, sounded, and felt like the demons that were controlling too many aspects of my life and to turn them into expressions of understanding and being understood.

I can't say whether those weeks on the ward gave rise to the seminal moment that helped me find a new way forward with my voice hearing. I had decided that I wasn't powerful enough on my own to deal with my day-to-day voices and visions. The peculiar sensations and beliefs that I was evil enough to harm others by contamination were too much. I knew about the principles of recovery as they were understood at the time my voices emerged. As a psychotherapist, I had a reasonable knowledge of how humans respond to distressing events. It is hard to say how helpful or hindering this knowledge was to begin with. My threat system was ignited in a way that made my thinking freeze and blocked my capacity to reflect. My coping strategy was primitive: running and walking miles was both literal and symbolic of my desire to escape these voices and what hearing them meant within a pathologising system. I was busy reacting to the moment and the only way I could respond to my professional knowledge about human distress was to feel utterly ashamed for not being able to apply it to myself and to have fallen into "psychosis" in the first place. So, initially, my decision to try and understand my voices and to not have my life managed by psychiatric services was constantly confounded by the shame and guilt I felt in response to what voices said and the state of my life as it was.

My decision to try and find a different way to understand and manage my voices didn't change anything about my voice hearing except the places I went looking for answers and solutions. There wasn't a single point in time when things changed. It was more a case of a growing and deepening understanding that changing the relationship with voices needed to become a pivotal "mechanism". I slowly grew in confidence to approach my voices. I started to become curious about them out of desperation and because running away and medicating myself into a stupor didn't work. I suspended my disbelief and started talking with one voice in particular, after learning this technique through a voice dialogue training workshop (we discuss this method later in this book). Slowly I gained more insight, more confidence, became more familiar with each voice. I got to know them. They were all difficult to engage with and I had many occasions of feeling like giving up, but glimmers of change and noticing a reduction in their hostility helped me keep going. The more I have worked directly with my voices, the easier it has become to live with my voices and live with myself.

At the time of writing, I still have challenging relationships with some voices. They can still scare and overwhelm me at times but less and less. I now have excellent relationships with a couple of my voices and a growing respect for and harmony with others. Four have not spoken at all for several years. I have found some very strong allies among a few voices to help me relate to my more difficult voices.

Everyone's voice hearing experience is different and unique. In making connections with other voice hearers and people who accept me, voices, and all, I found a way of wading through the distress and confusion and establishing a greater understanding of who my voices are and what they represent. Along that path I have found a way of first learning, then sharing pieces of knowledge and experience that have helped me and so help to write this book with no other intention than to help a voice hearer and the person who wants to help them. It is not a straightforward path, but I have found that a balance of establishing a sense of safety followed by a foray into the territory of a difficult voice, using curiosity, and a bit of bravery helps me to understand what my voices are about, who they are, and what they are trying to communicate, which is always, ultimately, once I can decode their messages, protective.

Having outlined how common voice hearing is and how it can be experienced, in the next chapter, we explore the bigger picture by setting out a broad sociopolitical context in which voice hearing has come to be understood and subsequently perceived as requiring treatment.

Chapter 2

The bigger picture

Mental healthcare "treatment" of voice hearing

Historically, voice hearing has been considered an unintelligible sign of madness. Even until relatively recent times, practitioners have been discouraged from engaging in discussion with patients about their voices for fear of collusion and making the situation worse. Even up to the present day, in mainstream mental healthcare, voices are framed as a symptom of an illness or disorder such as schizophrenia, which would typically become chronic and treated with drugs that have been marketed as a remedy to fix or cure the illness (for example, "anti" psychotic, anti-depressant, anxiolytic medication). There was an injection of hope during the 1990s following research evidence of successful applications of psychosocial approaches to support people diagnosed with schizophrenia. This initially included predominantly behavioural approaches but soon incorporated cognitive theory and also included the seminal work of Romme and Escher, which focused on accepting and establishing personal meaning associated with voices through making sense of how difficult life experiences might have contributed to voices. In the United Kingdom, there was also hope during this time following the reform and investment in public healthcare by the New Labour government from 1997. New policies led to the development of new mental health services, especially in the community, that focused on people who experienced psychosis or diagnosed with schizophrenia (many of whom heard voices). However, neoliberalism had begun to take effect on our healthcare services in terms of shaping how mental health broadly and voice hearing specifically were conventionally understood and subsequently "treated" by medication. This influenced an approach to understanding and "treating" mental health broadly and voice hearing specifically that focused on the individual and their internal factors rather than how that individual engaged in and was affected by their wider societal contexts. Global events such as the banking crisis during the late 2000s and COVID-19 in early 2020 negatively impacted society broadly and the provision of healthcare.

In this chapter, we flesh out this historical context and explore the bigger picture in relation to voice hearing. We outline some key issues relating to the broader sociopolitical context, which influences how our lives are governed and shapes the decisions governments make concerning our health and the extent to which support for our health is provided by the welfare state.

DOI: 10.4324/9781032619910-3

Medicalisation and pathologisation of voice hearing

There has been a long-standing debate between biomedical and psychosocial explanations regarding mental health distress, including voice hearing, with the former conceptualising voice hearing as a symptom of a dysfunctional brain and the latter conceptualising it as a reaction to psychosocial factors related to individual life experiences (Cooke, Smythe, & Anscombe, 2019; Shorter, 1998). For several decades, however, a prevailing biomedical disease narrative, certainly in Western psychiatry, has influenced the construction of an evidence base from which distressing experiences such as voice hearing have been understood (Johnstone & Boyle, 2018). According to Nettleton (2021), the biomedical model is based upon the following six assumptions: (1) the mind and body can be treated separately; (2) symptoms of illness or dysfunctional parts can be mended; (3) medicine adopts a "technological imperative"; (4) biological explanations of disease are reductive and marginalise other factors (i.e. psychological, sociological, cultural, etc.); (5) diseases are caused by a specific, identifiable "disease entity"; and (6) it is objective and universalised. In other words, the biological model pathologises emotional distress (including voice hearing) as a distinct mental illness (Johnstone & Boyle, 2018). Consequently, a biomedical explanation conceptualises health-related problems as a deviation from normal functioning and marginalises specific experiences such as voice hearing from personally meaningful and individual accounts.

Influence of sociopolitical context on health and healthcare

Readers might consider there to be parallels between this conventional approach and the dominant neoliberal discourse that threads through much of our society. Neoliberalism is a dominant ideology that has permeated public policies in terms of its emphasis on the "reduction of state intervention in economic and social activities and the deregulation of labor [sic] and financial markets" (Navarro, 2007). It is sometimes referred to as late capitalism and is argued to be "a distinctive political theory…[which]…holds that a society's political and economic institutions should be robustly liberal and capitalist, but supplemented by a constitutionally limited democracy and a modest welfare state" (Stanford Encyclopedia of Philosophy).

In recent years, scholars have been interested in exploring how neoliberal ideology has impacted understandings of mental health and subsequent mental healthcare practice (e.g., Davies, 2021; Davies, Pace, & Devenot, 2023; Esposito & Perez, 2014). James Davies refers to several structural elements within our societies that influence how we are governed and impact how we live and, consequently, how we make sense of and respond to health and distress. Davies and colleagues (Davies, 2021; Davies, Pace, & Devenot, 2023) have argued that conventional mental health treatments have aligned with several core mechanisms of neoliberalism, which have impacted health and healthcare. We can also relate this to voice hearing. These concern processes by which human phenomena (i.e., the way we think, our emotions, the actions we take, the physical experiences we recognise) are conceptualised within a medical framework (referred to as medicalisation) and subsequently pathologised to require medical intervention (pathologisation); or conceptualised in ways that avoid implicating the economy from contributing to individual suffering (depoliticisation); or for suffering to be reconceptualised into marketing opportunities from which money, and lots of it, can be made (commodification); and in ways that locate in the individual self the causes of suffering rather than broader societal or sociological explanations (de-collectivism or individualisation). As such, for many people distressed by voice hearing, typically their experience is one in which they have received one of the expanding number of diagnoses (most likely schizophrenia), which infers their distress has been medically framed and pathologised, the cause of which is predominantly if not exclusively rooted in their self and exclusive of wider societal influence, and thereby favouring change in themselves rather than their wider community or sociological context. Consequently, the current conventional approach favours individual rather than social reform so that the individual becomes more resilient to cope with broader societal conditions.

Returning to the medicalisation and pathologisation of voice hearing

Informed by these neoliberal core mechanisms, the prevailing understanding of voice hearing has been informed by an overemphasis on locating the causation and maintenance of voice hearing in the individual self, which has marginalised broader sociological factors (e.g., culture, political, etc.) within which voice hearing is experienced. For example, when a person distressed by voice hearing is admitted to mental healthcare, they typically receive a diagnosis such as schizophrenia, which is part of a powerful biomedical disease narrative about the nature and cause of voice hearing that typically marginalises more personally meaningful narratives. Aligned with neoliberal values, there has been increased emphasis on individualism and free market competition shaping decisions about healthcare. The classification of mental health distress as an illness, disorder, or disease has been shaped by political and/or profit-driven objectives associated with commodifying medicalisation of life experiences and a proliferation of individualised medication treatments with a rationale to treat biomedical illnesses (and benefitting pharmaceutical companies) (Esposito & Perez, 2014).

So, according to the biomedical approach, voice hearing is a symptom of an illness (typically schizophrenia), which is assumed to be caused by biochemical, neuroendocrine, structural, and genetic abnormalities in the brain (Andreasen, 1985). This assumes that explanatory causes of voice hearing are predominantly internal and genetically predetermined, i.e. voices are due to a person's dysfunctional brain. Consequently, this approach informs practitioners to investigate for, and prescribe treatment to target, the biological causes of symptoms of health-related problems. Potential underlying problems beyond the voice hearer's internal world are considered less relevant and disregarded. As such, personal narratives that potentially link emotional distress with adverse life experiences within wider social, cultural, political, and economic contexts are marginalised. This can lead to a belief that people who hear voices are passive victims of a mental disease and impact an individual's agency, identity and the meaning they might ascribe to personal and distressing experiences (Johnstone & Boyle, 2018). It is important to note, however, that despite the dominance and general acceptance of this perspective of mental health distress broadly and voice hearing specifically, no biological markers for diagnoses such as schizophrenia (and specifically for experiences such as voice hearing) have been identified. Furthermore, research evidence that supports this perspective has been critiqued by numerous scholars to have been beset with methodological flaws based on poor reporting methods, poor and inconsistent diagnostic criteria, and over-inclusion of a wide spectrum of diagnostic disorders, lack of blinding (researchers) and comparison group, and artificial inflation of the genetic contribution (e.g., Fleming & Martin, 2011).

Conventional mainstream approaches to "treat" voice hearing

Informed by the biomedical model, following admission to mental healthcare, typically a person's distress is medically framed, pathologised and the support provided is framed as treatment. The general aim of this treatment is to eradicate underlying factors that cause the distress, i.e., voice hearing, or at least to reduce the voice hearing. Recommended treatment approaches include "antipsychotic" medication and psychological therapy (which includes Cognitive Behavioural Therapy [CBT], Family Intervention, Art Therapies, and although not recommended, it is recognised that other therapies such as counselling, supportive psychotherapy, and social skills training might be preferential for some people) (NICE, 2014). However, there has been long-standing debate within academic literature regarding the most effective way to treat voice hearing. Furthermore, there is also a question in terms of what such treatment should address. For example, should treatment focus on an approach to eradicate or reduce the voice hearing or improve the experience of hearing voices? Some people who hear voices do not believe their voices need to be treated or removed, but some people do. We first summarise mainstream treatment approaches below before we consider some alternative approaches that have become available for people distressed by voice hearing.

Antipsychotic medication

Antipsychotic medication is the primary first-line intervention for difficulties related to mental health broadly and for voice hearing specifically (e.g., NICE, 2014). It is prescribed as a treatment for most people distressed by voice hearing (e.g., McManus, Bebbington, Jenkins, & Brugha, 2016). However, people can have complex relationships with medication. We will consider this further in Part 2 when we explore the development of the Tripartite Relationship Theory, but for now, we want to highlight that there are mixed perceptions and experiences concerning medication. Some people believe they benefit from using antipsychotic medication, some do not. Indeed, some people simultaneously believe they benefit from using it but also believe they are harmed by it. Whilst we wish to respect all individual preferences and experiences of using medication, we believe the most important element for people taking it is for them to have informed choice. Genuine choice. And for individuals to have the agency to exercise their choice. In other words, we believe it is most important for individuals to be able to make their own decisions about whether to use medication. This is also something we will return to throughout this book in terms of the level of agency a person has, not just with regard to their voice hearing experiences but also concerning their involvement and decisions regarding their own support and treatment.

Unfortunately, the dominant role of medication and the way in which it is used in mental healthcare cause us concern. To briefly return to one of the core mechanisms of neoliberalism, commodification has involved the marketing and subsequent prominent role of antipsychotic medication as a treatment and the large profits they bring for pharmaceutical companies. Indeed, the term "antipsychotic" is nothing more than effective marketing. The number of prescriptions has continually increased in recent years, despite concerns regarding the evidence underlying the use of these medications (such as unreliable or missing data reported by pharmaceutical companies, statistical and methodological flaws and poor study design, and publication bias overestimating efficacy (Sharma, Guski, Freund, & Gøtzsche, 2016; Driessen, Hollon, Bockting, Cuijpers, & Turner, 2015; Goldacre, 2014; Goldacre, 2010; Bentall, 2009; Moncrieff, 2008).

Generally, research evidence suggests that the use of antipsychotic medication is more effective than placebo (in other words, compared to a pretend equivalent drug) in the short term only. For example, a systematic review in 2020 found that, even accounting for poor reporting of randomisation, allocation, and blinding, antipsychotics are more effective than placebo in preventing relapse and reducing hospitalisation over a period of less than 12 months (Ceraso et al., 2020). Evidence supporting longer term use of medication, however, is contested. A criticism of the research evidence supporting the use of antipsychotic medication is that most trials typically last for only short periods of time, often under 12 weeks. In contrast, there have been at least eight studies by eight different groups of researchers who have found no benefits with longer term use (7–20 years) of antipsychotic medication (Harrow, Jobe, Faull, & Yang, 2017; Kotov et al., 2017; Morgan et al., 2017; Wils et al., 2017; Moilanen et al., 2013; Harrison et al., 2001; Bland & Parker, 1978). Additionally, unwanted side effects from taking these medications are commonly reported and there are many studies evidencing the harm, which has been acknowledged in the National Institute for Health and Clinical Excellence (NICE) guidelines for several years.

Policy shaping healthcare support for voice hearing

The development of the current conventional approach to understanding and responding to mental health distress, including voice hearing, has taken place within a sociopolitical context in which health policy and research evidence have influenced and shaped healthcare service provision.

Despite the long-standing debate and concern related to the effectiveness and harms associated with antipsychotic medication, typically almost without exception, individuals admitted to mental health services due to voice-related distress are in receipt of it as a treatment. The UK mental healthcare comprises a network of inpatient and community services, in which primary care General Practitioner (GP) services act as a first point of access for most people. There are numerous providers, the largest of which is the National Health Service (NHS). Most of the standard care is provided by the NHS, and specifically by community services and, when sufficient support for acute distress is unable to be provided, acute inpatient services that can provide intensive, short-term treatment (Simpson, Allison, & Lambley, 2017). There are also alternative forms of mental health services (e.g., see Johnson et al., 2009) that are fewer in number and generally provide support for people exhibiting less disturbed behaviour. As such, generally, distress related to voice hearing is more likely to be treated in standard NHS services.

Over the last three decades, there has been significant change in the provision of mental healthcare. The National Framework for Mental Health was the first of several ambitious mental health policies introduced by the then New Labour government from the late 1990s. This was a long-term strategy to invest in the mental healthcare workforce and drive up the quality of mental healthcare (Thornicroft, 2000), which included psychological therapies. Initially, the focus for change was on community services, with details set out in 2000 in The NHS Plan for three new specialist community services relevant to people distressed by voice hearing: Assertive Outreach Teams (for people whom mental health service had historically struggled or failed to engage), Crisis Resolution Teams (to support people in an acute crisis), and Early Intervention Teams (to support people experiencing early signs of psychosis for the first time). These services have since evolved but continue to remain central to current mental healthcare provision.

Around the same time, in 1999, a new executive non-departmental public body of the Department of Health in England, the NICE, was established with a remit to produce treatment guidance for practitioners based on the best available evidence. Over time, NICE evolved to become the National Institute for Health and Clinical Excellence (in 2005) and then the National Institute for Health and Care Excellence (in 2013). The first clinical guideline was published in 2002 and concerned schizophrenia, which was replaced in 2009 with an increasingly broader focus on psychosis and schizophrenia, and further updated again in 2014 to the current version (NICE, 2014). The guidelines have increasingly recognised the importance of psychological therapy, specifically CBT, as a treatment for psychosis, including voice hearing. Shortly following the introduction of NSF-MH, the NHS Plan, and

NICE, there was renewed focus on improving the quality of mental health inpatient healthcare through the 2002 Mental Health Policy Implementation Guide: Adult Acute Inpatient Care Provision. A key focus of this guide was to maximise the quality of practitioners' therapeutic time with patients and to include patients in treatment decision-making.

Although these policies brought much-needed investment and reform to mental healthcare, disaster struck a few years later in 2008 with the global banking crisis, which required governments to step in with public money to bail out financial institutions. Compounding the impact of this on public services, including healthcare, this was subsequently followed by a period of austerity, which was implemented in the United Kingdom two years later by the then Conservative/Liberal Democrat Coalition Government, to reduce the budget deficit in response to the effects of the banking crisis. The detrimental effects of this were soon observed in healthcare services constrained by the long shadow of austerity measures (and have stretched to present-day mental healthcare provision). For example, a particularly significant change came with the Health and Social Care Act 2012 that transferred the commissioning of healthcare to groups of GPs in Clinical Commissioning Groups (in England) but led to concerns regarding cost-cutting and how the commissioning process could increase patient choice whilst facilitate competition (e.g. if GPs consider medication as a front-line treatment for mental health rather than the limited availability of psychological therapies, patient choice is compromised) (Glover-Thomas, 2013). There was also explicit recognition in the 2014 NHS Five Year Forward View of a "funding and efficiency gap" (p. 7) that posed a risk to quality care and staffing resources, and a political signal that "the economic prosperity of Britain…depend[ed] on a radical upgrade in prevention and public health" (p. 3). This gave emphasis to public health and empowerment of individuals to be supported to manage their own health. This last point touches on one of the broader issues concerning neoliberalism introduced earlier. That is, mental distress (and specifically voice hearing) was rooted in the individual self both as cause and remedy, with much less recognition or value placed on potential factors external to the individual self.

An independent Commission shortly after the publication of the NHS Five Year Forward View revealed nationwide variation in the quality of mental health acute units, especially regarding the quality of treatment and concerns related to staff shortages, poor staff morale, and burnout (Crisp, Smith, & Nicholson, 2016). It was then acknowledged in the 2016 Five Year Forward View for Mental Health that there had been insufficient provision of NICE-recommended treatment for patients, including long waits for people with severe mental health problems for psychological therapies (or not even having access at all). The huge cuts to public and welfare spending during this period of austerity disproportionately affected the health and well-being of vulnerable groups and mental health services (British Medical Association, 2016). A systematic narrative review of the health effects of the economic crisis in high-income countries later found that mental health had been the most adversely affected by it (Karanikolos, Heino, McKee, Stuckler, & Legido-Quigley, 2016).

The NHS Long Term Plan (NHS, 2019) renewed a commitment to grow investment in mental health services faster than the NHS budget overall, which included a commitment of at least an additional £2.3bn on mental healthcare, increased provision of psychological therapies for depression and anxiety and community-based physical and mental healthcare for people with severe mental illness, all by 2023/2024. However, some 12 years on from the global bank crisis, there was further global disaster. On 11th March 2020, the World Health Organisation (WHO) declared the COVID-19 pandemic. Healthcare and economies suffered globally, with the effects still felt to the present day and most likely for many years to come. In addition to the devastating impact on the mortality and morbidity of the global population, practitioners reported increased levels of stress, depression, suicide, burnout, and mental exhaustion (Fiorillo & Gorwood, 2020) and raised concerns regarding scarcity of resources and effective treatment options (Heale & Wray, 2020). For many people, their face-to-face contact with healthcare practitioners was reduced during stricter periods of the pandemic and replaced by alternative methods such as telemedicine.

Throughout the publication of healthcare policies such as those mentioned above, and the impact of global disasters such as the banking crisis and Covid-19, the influence of neoliberal core mechanisms can be observed. Mental distress broadly, and voice hearing specifically, had been medically framed, pathologised, and treated predominantly with increasing amounts of prescribed medication. Even with more recent recognition of psychological therapy, this has been typically considered to be an adjunct to medication. Some people distressed by voice hearing receive psychotherapy, albeit following a lengthy waiting list, but almost without exception, all people are prescribed psychotropic medication. There has been insufficient recognition in health-related policy and mental healthcare provision of wider societal influences on mental distress or specific concerns related to voice hearing.

The above summary of some of the developments concerning mental healthcare and the impact of key global events on these illustrates the considerable changes to service provision of mental health support. Laudable aims of numerous policies have included increases to the range of mental health service provision and increases to the choice of treatments within these services. However, despite these ambitions, a gap exists between the targets set out in policy and the real-world clinical experiences in mental healthcare. Patients are becoming more acutely unwell at the point of hospital admission, more likely to be diagnosed with psychosis (and troubled by voice hearing) and of higher risk (Gilburt, 2015; McCrone, Dhanasiri, Patel, Knapp, & Lawton-Smith, 2008). However, chronic underinvestment in mental health services has led to concerning levels of inequality of service provision and services under increasing financial pressures (British Medical Association, 2016; Gilburt, 2015; Foley, 2013). The increasing financial pressure has constrained the provision of recommended evidence-based mental health treatment. Reduced funding to mental health services has led to insufficient community services, a reduction of inpatient beds, and inpatient services treating patients with increased levels of distress (Gilburt, 2015). Additionally, an increasingly generic, non-registered, non-specialist, and junior workforce has been challenged with delivering evidence-based treatment (Gilburt, 2015).

Although our portrayal of the above broader sociopolitical backdrop has considered only a selection of key policy and developments, we believe there is wide agreement that mental health practitioners have been at breaking point for some time due to prolonged understaffing and increasing demand on services, with the British Medical Association calling for the UK Government to ensure mental healthcare receives equitable resources as physical healthcare (Mahase, 2020). Consequently, despite the intentions and recommendations set out in policy regarding investment in mental health services, austerity and chronic underfunding have negatively impacted mental health services. Unsurprisingly, these services have struggled under sustained pressure. This has contributed to pressure on inpatient and community services, insufficient provision for individuals in crisis, increased use of the Mental Health Act, and pressures on practitioners who are expected to do more but with less resource (Cummins, 2018). Consequently, mental health practitioners increasingly struggle to sufficiently support and treat people, including voice hearers, with acute mental health problems.

It is within this broader context that mental healthcare has developed in recent years, and in which support for people distressed by voice hearing has been made available. We first summarise the standard approaches provided for people before we turn to less conventional alternatives to standard healthcare provision.

Against the neoliberal backdrop and global events referred to above, and in addition to the increasing amount of medication usage, there have also been promising developments in psychosocial approaches. Despite the prolific use of antipsychotic medication as a form of treatment for people distressed by voice hearing, unfortunately they do not provide individuals with an increased understanding of their voice hearing. Taking antipsychotic medication does not lead an individual to develop an understanding of why they hear voices, why *their specific* voices, what the voices say, what role they have in the individual's life, and what might become of their voices in the future. Medication also does not have the ability to change the circumstances in which the person experiences their voice hearing. However, learning and understanding about voice hearing experiences is important for recovery for many people.

CBT for psychosis

In addition to antipsychotic medication, people distressed by voice hearing might also be offered a form of psychological support known as CBT. This is a trauma-informed form of talking therapy (Hardy et al., 2023) that has developed from extensive research over several decades and across a wide range of health conditions. It is hypothesised that trauma influences the development of beliefs and/ or increases a person's vulnerability and susceptibility to hearing voices or developing psychosis. It has been adapted specifically for people experiencing psychosis and/or voice hearing, referred to as CBT for psychosis (or CBTp). From the first adaptation to psychosis from Chadwick and Birchwood (1994) and the research of many other scholars, it is hypothesised according to the CBTp model that, rather than the content of what a voice(s) might say, it is what voice hearers belief(s) about their voice(s) and specifically regarding the power, purpose, and identity of them, which causes distress for individuals and influences how they respond to their voice(s). The CBTp approach concerns power relations between the individual and their voices and the control they have over their voices (e.g. Birchwood & Chadwick, 1997; Mawson, Berry, Murray, & Hayward, 2011; Rácz, Kaló, Kassai, Kiss, & Pintér, 2017). Essentially, the CBTp approach hypothesises that individuals who hear voices undergo a perceptual error of some sort, for example they misattribute a sound or experience and conclude it to be a voice. As such, the focus of therapy concerns their appraisals and subsequent meaning-making regarding their voices.

Interestingly, although CBTp is the most widely available psychological talking therapy for voice hearing, it has received criticism. For example, some have argued that in focusing on beliefs, insufficient attention has been given to help people understand core reasons why they hear voices (McCarthy-Jones & Longden, 2013); only a small effect size has been found on overall "symptoms" (Jauhar et al., 2014; Garety et al., 2008), which means little difference has been found in trials between CBTp when compared to standard care; there is only preliminary evidence specifically for voices that issue commands, clinically referred to as command hallucinations (Pontillo et al., 2016); it is costly to provide large-scale training, which means only small segments of the workforce are able to deliver it, and consequently, it is difficult to make it consistently widely available (Thomas et al., 2014).

Romme and Escher and the Hearing Voices Movement: linking life history and voice hearing

At around the same time as CBT-informed therapies for psychosis began to evolve, so too did an approach that would eventually come to be referred to as the Maastricht approach, developed through the seminal work of Marius Romme and Sandra Escher. In the 1980s, psychiatrist Romme treated a young woman, Patsy Hage, who had been distressed by voice hearing. When Romme referred to her voices as a symptom of a biomedical illness, Hage challenged his belief as reductionist and questioned how he could believe in a God he hadn't seen or heard, yet not believe voice hearing as nothing more than a symptom of a disease. Romme later reflected on the unhelpfulness of his biomedical framing and subsequent medication for Hage's voice hearing. So, with help from Escher, a researcher trained in journalism (and married to Romme), they approached and appeared on a Dutch national television talk show where Hage told her story about her voice hearing. They asked the viewers to contact them if they knew how to cope with voices and 700 people responded. They returned a questionnaire to those who responded and 450 people returned it, of which 150 reported they were able to cope with their voices, and some were even happy to hear them, without any involvement of psychiatry. From this, Romme and Escher concluded that voice hearing per se isn't problematic; rather it is the *experience* of it that can be the problem. A year later, the first Hearing Voices Congress was held in the Netherlands, which subsequently grew into a global voice hearing movement that spread first to the United Kingdom and then widely across Europe, Australia, the United States, and beyond.

This provided a platform for people to share their experiences of hearing voices and to challenge conventional ideology in psychiatry for the right for people to define their own experiences. Romme and Escher (Romme, Escher, Dillon, Corstens, & Morris, 2009; Romme & Escher, 2000; Romme & Escher, 1993) stressed the importance of accepting voices as real, rather than a meaningless symptom of an illness or disease and later with colleagues (Romme et al, 2009) made several recommendations for practitioners to reduce stigma and isolation related to voice hearing: (1) accepting voices as real, which places emphasis on an individual's frame of reference to interpret and make personal meaning rather than impose professional frameworks; (2) the importance of understanding the language used by voices, e.g., voices might communicate using metaphors such as referring to light and dark to represent love and hate rather than interpreting their words in a literal sense; (3) helping individuals to communicate with their voices (see further discussion below regarding the Talking with Voices [TwV] approach and AVATAR therapy); (4) encouraging people who hear voices to meet with other voice hearers.

The work of Romme and Escher emphasised the association between life experiences, voice hearing, and the impact of relationships on voice hearing. From their work, and subsequent work of others they inspired, voice hearing is best understood as a reaction to problems in life and between people. They theorised three distinct phases of voice hearing, a pattern many voice hearers recognise: the Startle Phase (shock and chaos), the Organisation Phase (accepting, understanding and finding meaning), and the Stabilisation Phase (reclaiming power and living with voices). Rather than a linear move from chaos towards a greater sense of order and stable voice hearing experiences, setbacks and progress can happen at different times for voice hearers. It can be helpful for voice hearers, practitioners and supporters to be aware of these phases of voice hearing as a way of understanding where the voice hearer is on their journey.

Startle phase

This initial phase tends to be characterised by bewilderment, fear, and a loss of control. Typically, when someone starts to hear voices that are distressing, the experience is shocking. It can be so destabilising and frightening that a person cannot trust what is and is not real, cannot even trust the ground they walk on. In terms of what voices say, if it is disturbing, it can re-awaken previous traumatic experiences. Voices can speak directly about those difficult experiences. The nature of the content of voices is usually very personal. It can feel like being haunted by past experiences the voice hearer would rather forget. RL's first experience of voice hearing felt like being forced to listen to soundtracks and watch videos of her worst experiences without being able to turn them off even in her sleep. They were terrifying and paralysing, with a sense that there was no escape.

When first starting to hear distressing voices, the level of shock, fear, and questioning of reality causes many voice hearers to find ways of trying to escape the voices. They might try to keep the experience to themselves, self-isolate, or seek prescribed or illicit drugs to numb or silence their voices. They may put on a "brave face" to hide distress, self-injure (including binging or purging food) to numb the distress. This phase is often marked by both attempts to quell the distress in any way that seems feasible and at the same time to try and make meaning and understand what is happening to them and who they have become.

Organisation phase

Many voice hearers gradually find their own way of moving into a more organised place with their voices. This can happen through several means, including recognising predictable triggers that may help the voice hearer protect themselves; voices may spontaneously or gradually fade or become silent; changes to life circumstances that help build self-confidence and self-esteem; becoming more familiar and knowledgeable about voices; finding meaningful things to do that bring purpose, distraction from voices and enjoyment; forming trusting and supportive relationships; attending Hearing Voices Groups; and engaging in talking therapies.

Stabilisation phase

As a voice hearer finds more ways of organising, tolerating, and working with voices, they may develop more helpful relationships and meaningful occupations outside of direct voice management. This can allow more opportunities to find ways of living more peacefully with their voices in ways that suit who they are and their beliefs. The nature of the ups and downs in life means that people are constantly offered different developmental experiences that can help move a person forward. Putting oneself slightly outside a comfort zone can help build confidence and resilience beneficial for managing voices. Voice hearers and voices may become less distressed because of the voice hearer initiating their self-agency by doing meaningful activities that are specific to their personal interests and values, and thus growing a breadth to their life in a healthy way. This helps a voice hearer move towards the stabilisation phase and can make them feel more stable with some capacity to resist the messages from voices and perhaps others that seem to deny their rights to confidence and a good life. Equally, challenging experiences can destabilise and cause them to revisit previous phases. For example, the death of someone important or the break-up of an important relationship can be distressing and perhaps disturb voices at a time when one is less able to modulate strong feelings and negative, critical messages. It could feel like being thrown back into the original chaos. Taking time to re-stabilise and reconnect gently with voices and the world allows voices to settle as they accommodate to life. It also gives time to pull out useful learning about themselves and voices.

The stabilisation phase doesn't mean that voice hearers get to a constant state of equilibrium with their voices and cease to be impacted by them. Instead, they become more knowledgeable about themselves and who the voices are, and more accepting of the voices and so able to swing with the upward and downward swoops of life. Giving oneself permission to take time to re-stabilise if thrown off balance is critical. Recovery does not necessarily have an endpoint. Voices may always have something new to say and finding the wisdom within these transactions is one of the keys to moving forward.

Romme and Escher's early work also led to the development of the Hearing Voices Movement, which holds six core values (Corstens, Longden, McCarthy-Jones, Waddingham, & Thomas, 2014): (1) voices are normalised as a common human experience; (2) they are also framed as an understandable response to life events; (3) diverse explanations for them are valued, including biomedical; (4) the importance of owning and defining one's own voice hearing experience; (5) support from other people who hear voices to help make sense of and cope with one's own is valued; (6) accepting and valuing voices as real.

These values are at odds with the neoliberal core mechanisms and mainstream mental healthcare, described earlier in this chapter. This is an alternative approach to the conventional treatment provided in mental healthcare but advocates for personal meaning related to problems in living and interpreted by the individual in relation to their life history and, as such, is rooted in the interaction between individuals and their societal contexts.

Lack of choice and control: a focus on containment

However, within this neoliberal context of policy-driven service development and global events, mental healthcare has been criticised for lacking therapeutic quality and infringing human rights. Health policy and mental health law legitimise the control and restriction of patients' movement, and the enforcement of treatment even when unwanted. This relates to both hospital (or equivalent) and community settings. Commonly referred to as coercion, patients can be persuaded to accept treatment or to do something by the issue of a threat or force. Coercive practice has been acknowledged as a global concern by the World Psychiatric Association (Kallert, Monahan, & Mezzich, 2007). This is to the extent that the WHO has raised concerns regarding the violation of human rights against patients, including those distressed by voice hearing (https://www.who.int/news-room/fact-sheets/detail/schizophrenia).

Although NICE (2015) recommends the use of restrictive interventions only if other de-escalation and preventative approaches have failed and non-action presents as a risk to the patient and/or other people, rising levels of coercion in mental health services have been recognised in numerous reports (e.g., Modernising the Mental Health Act (Department of health and Social Care), 2018; CQC, 2011, 2013, 2014, 2015, 2016, 2017). In addition to the widespread use of coercion, there is also a lack of genuine choice for people admitted to mental healthcare. For example, as we discussed earlier in this chapter, recommended treatment for people distressed by voice hearing includes medication and psychological interventions (CQC, 2015; NICE, 2014). However, in real-world practice, this choice is largely restricted to only medication (The Commission on Acute Adult Psychiatric Care, 2015; CQC, 2017). Insufficient access to evidence-based treatment such as CBTp (Gilburt, 2015) and a postcode lottery to treatment (CQC, 2017) result in patients' needs, including voice hearers, being insufficiently met. Furthermore, there have also been numerous reports that have raised concerns regarding the quality of care in mental health services. For example, the application of blanket rules that has included limited access to outside areas or internet access of restricted visiting times (CQC, 2014), as high 86% of doors locked wards that detain everyone in all but name and deny all patients their autonomy (CQC, 2013) and an increased use of Community Treatment Orders (CQC, 2015). As such, mental healthcare comprises a "control and containment" culture with over-reliance on medication and a lack of personalised care (CQC, 2013).

Relationships

Throughout the last two decades, and challenging the conventional approach in mainstream mental healthcare, there has also been increasing interest to understand voice hearing as a relational experience that extends beyond the individual and their internal factors. Alongside and influenced by the development of psychological approaches, including the Maastricht approach, to understanding and supporting people experiencing distress related to voice hearing (or other experiences), attention also turned to investigate life experiences. In other words, contrary to an individual's internal experiences as an explanatory model advocated by the biomedical model, there has also been growing interest in exploring external factors such as traumatic events as potential factors contributing to distress (for example, voice hearing). As such, there is now good evidence of a correlation between difficult life experiences and voice hearing. Numerous research has shown that people who hear voices also report to have experienced one or more life events they believed were traumatic (Bentall & Varese, 2013; Read & Bentall, 2012; Varese et al., 2012; Lardinois, Lataster, Mengelers, Van Os, & MyinGermeys, 2011; Larkin & Read, 2008), including anxiety before and during voice hearing (Delespaul, de Vries, & van Os, 2002) and even bereavement (Kamp, O'Connor, Spindler, & Moskowitz, 2019). There has been increased interest in recent years in investigating links between psychosis (and specifically voice hearing) and trauma. Several studies have found that many people who hear voices report that traumatic experiences of some sort have led to the onset of their voice hearing (discussed below). This line of inquiry can provide important personal historical contexts related to hearing voices that might help explain underlying emotions associated with voices (Johnstone, 2009; Dillon, 2012).

We know from the literature and from our own experiences of working with people distressed by voice hearing that previous abusive experiences are often perceived as traumatic and can be represented in voice hearing, for example in the physical appearance, character, or sound (or a combination of all) of voices. Although not all people who hear voices have experienced trauma, and correlation does not equate to causation, many people with particularly distressing voices have experienced trauma (Luhrmann et al., 2019). The research evidence from trauma-related studies has significantly contributed to challenging the biomedical disease narrative concerning voice hearing. Increasingly, the potential contribution of a person's life history is recognised as significant to voice hearing experiences. It has also shaped the evolvement of psychological approaches to support people distressed by voice hearing, as we discuss below.

In placing importance on the relationship between individuals and their voices, Romme and Escher (1993, 2000) and colleagues (2009) argued that it is this relationship that determines whether an individual becomes distressed by their voice hearing. This is commonly acknowledged in contemporary psychosocial approaches to understand and support people distressed by voice hearing. Over the past 30 years, the focus of early CBT-informed psychological approaches that conceptualised voices as a sensory or thought-like stimulus, and which focused on individual beliefs about voices, evolved to conceptualise voices as social, person-like stimulus, and shifted the focus to consider how individuals relate with their voices (Hayward, Berry, McCarthy-Jones, Strauss, & Thomas, 2014; Hayward, 2003). This has contributed to a significant change in thinking about voice hearing. For many people, contrary to a disease narrative of biomedicine, treatment responses should not be concerned with getting rid of voices. Instead, it should be concerned with reducing distress related to voice hearing by changing the relationship between individuals and their voices and to support individuals to reclaim their power from voices (Romme et al., 2009, Romme and Escher, 2000, 1993). Our work aligns with this. We have also observed that voice-related distress is associated with difficulties individuals experience in terms of how they relate to their voices and their lack of perceived power in relation to their voices, which we will discuss in more detail in the next section of this book.

Romme et al. (2009, p. 9) states "voices are the stories of threatening emotions; emotions of the person twisted by terrible experiences, hopelessness, feelings of guilt, aggression and anxiety". Expanding on this, Corstens, Longden, and May (2012) assert that voices serve a protective function. This gives importance to understanding and developing helpful ways of relating with voices and, to help construct this, to learn how to communicate with voices. Included in the evolvement of psychosocial approaches to understanding and supporting distress related to voice hearing are two interesting approaches that are aligned with this relational framework: TwV and AVATAR therapy.

Talking with Voices

Rooted in the work of the Hearing Voices Movement, and influenced by Voice Dialogue (Stone & Stone, 1989), TwV is a communication method that aims to facilitate helpful ways of relating and integration between individuals and their voices. The Voice Dialogue approach aims to address relational difficulties through exploring and communicating different parts of oneself (Stone & Stone use the terms "parts", "energies", or "selves" interchangeably).

Many people communicate with their voices, perhaps during Hearing Voices Group meetings or when they are on their own; however, there is limited but growing research evidence supporting the utilisation of this approach (see Hardy et al., 2023 for further details). The evidence suggests this is a helpful approach for people to engage with, build more helpful relationships with, and make sense of their voices. It is also the approach that we practice, and we will come back to discuss this in more detail in Part 3 of this book. The approach opens up the opportunity for lines of helpful communication between an individual and their voices, which can be facilitated by a third party. A helper, family member, friend, etc. can engage in direct verbal communication with a voice through the voice hearer. The aim is to create harmony and facilitate a process of integration between the voice(s) and the voice hearer.

AVATAR therapy

Another relational approach that targets interpersonal relationship between a hearer and their distressing voices is AVATAR therapy. Developed by Julian Leff in the United Kingdom, this involves a visual and auditory simulation, represented by the development of a 2D visual embodiment of the voice. Similar to the TwV approach, this subsequently offers an opportunity for a face-to-face dialogue. The voice hearer can then talk to the avatar voice simulation, facilitated by a therapist. Similar to the TwV, the aim is for the voice hearer to feel empowered from the experience of dialogue and in their relationship with the voice. The research evidence suggests this is more helpful than supportive counselling and increased a sense of power and control over one's voice hearing (Craig et al., 2018). Delivered in two phases, the first aims to reduce anxiety and increase power and control related to the voices, and the second aims to develop personal meaning associated with the voice.

Positioning our work in this background context

Our approach builds on the psychological approaches of relational theory and Romme and Escher, but in addition to focusing on relationships with voices, we also include practitioners (or others) in a tripartite relational context. This leads us into Chapter 3 and Part 2, where we turn our attention to the theoretical approach underlying our discussion for the remainder of this book.

Part 2

Tripartite Relationship Theory

The background context described in Part 1 has significantly influenced our approach to thinking and making sense about voice hearing and supporting people distressed by voices. In Part 2 of this book, we introduce the Tripartite Relationship Theory (Allison, 2022), developed by one of us (Rob Allison (RA)) within this broader context. This provides a theoretical framework for the supportive approaches we discuss in Part 3. First, in this introduction to Part 2, we briefly describe the research approach undertaken to develop the theory.

To develop the Tripartite Relationship Theory, decisions were made regarding, first, how to study voice hearing and, second, how to develop the learning from the study into a theory. Regarding studying voice hearing, RA was specifically interested to understand voice hearing experiences within relationship and clinical contexts to help inform practitioners in their approaches to support people in mental healthcare when distressed by voice hearing. As such, RA met and had conversations about voice hearing and mental healthcare with people who had experiences of hearing voices and receiving mental healthcare. He also met with mental healthcare practitioners who provided support for people distressed by voice hearing. In terms of collecting, analysing, and making sense of the information from these conversations, a methodological approach commonly utilised in the social sciences and healthcare research called Grounded Theory (more on this shortly) was chosen. We provide an overview of the approach taken to develop the Tripartite Relationship Theory in this section before discussing in more detail the experiences of voice hearers and practitioners and, finally, we explain how these experiences are represented within a relational context of voice hearer-voice practitioner.

The science behind the Tripartite Relationship Theory

In this section, we describe the research process undertaken to develop the theory. Broadly, research can be defined as either quantitative, qualitative, or a mix of both. Quantitative research is an approach suitable for examining causal or correlational relationships between different measurable variables and deductively generates knowledge about phenomena. For example, from investigating whether feeling lonely or socially isolated increases the amount of hostility experienced from

DOI: 10.4324/9781032619910-4

voices, we might conclude that maintaining regular social relationships reduces the amount of distress experienced by voice hearers. By contrast, qualitative research is an approach suitable for examining in-depth meaning and understanding within specific contexts and inductively generates knowledge about phenomena. For example, investigating a person's experience of voice hearing during their interactions with family and friends might help us learn more about how voices communicate to voice hearers during social settings. A mixture of both quantitative and qualitative approaches, also known as mixed methods, is an increasingly common approach in health-related research. Given the aim of the research was to explore, in depth, the experiences of voice hearing for people in mental healthcare, a qualitative approach was suitable.

The study was designed to explore voice hearing experiences and involved two stages. The first stage involved interviewing 15 people who heard voices and had received support from mental health services in relation to their voice hearing. We will discuss this in more detail in the next chapter. Following these interviews, the second stage involved interviewing a total of 18 mental health practitioners across 3 different focus groups. We will also come back to discuss this in more detail in Chapter 4. The different perspectives and experiences from the interviews with voice hearers and from the focus groups with practitioners were then synthesised, or brought together, to complete the development of the Tripartite Relationship Theory. We will examine this in more detail in Chapter 5.

Before we go into these details, however, we first provide a brief overview of the approach taken to conduct the research. To proceed with any research study, a research methodology must be chosen to provide the overarching strategy, or systematic approach, to generate knowledge during the research and in which specific research methods (i.e., interviews or focus groups) are utilised to collect and analyse information. Grounded Theory is a commonly utilised research methodology suitable for investigating phenomena, in which there is a clear process to collect and analyse data (i.e., experiences of voice hearing) and to develop theory (Birks & Mills, 2015; Charmaz, 2014). There are several versions that, according to Charmaz (2017), share the following common features: (1) an aim to develop theory that is specifically grounded in the research data, i.e., the experiences of hearing voices or the experiences of trying to support people who hear voices; (2) focus on patterns in the research data rather than focus on individual stories, i.e., focus on commonalities across the range of information from the interviews/focus groups from different voice hearers/practitioners rather than one individual person; (3) analysis of the information a person shares (i.e., about their voices) as soon as it is collected and before going on to interview other people rather than waiting until all the research data is collected before analysing it (known as concurrent data collection and analysis); (4) the analysis (as described in the previous point) informs decisions about who to interview next or from where to collect further information (known as theoretical sampling); (5) constant checking regarding how the analysis of the information compares with other analysed information, i.e. comparing what an individual says in one point of an interview with what they have said at other points in the interview, and also comparing what they have said against what other interviewees have said (known as constant comparison); (6) focus on actions and processes when analysing the information, i.e., being interested in patterns of behaviour or underlying social processes associated with voice hearing; and (7) the researcher to record their reflections of the research and subsequent analysis throughout the study (known as memo writing). This structured approach and clear focus on developing theory grounded in the experiences of voice hearers and practitioners made this a suitable methodology for the study.

However, notwithstanding the commonalities noted above regarding the different versions of Grounded Theory methodology, it was necessary to select a specific version for the study. The main difference between these several versions concerns the philosophical assumptions of the researcher (Mills, Bonner, & Francis, 2006) and it was at this point that a decision on which version to select was made. Charmaz's assertion that research provides "an interpretive portrayal of the studied world, not an exact picture of it" (Charmaz, 2014, p 17), and her acknowledgement of the researcher's "subjectivity and the researcher's involvement in the construction and interpretation of data" (p 14), aligns our worldview of multiple interpretations of voice hearing with Charmaz's constructive version of Grounded Theory. From our experiences, we believe that different people who hear voices develop a range of different understandings of their voice hearing experiences, and these can change or evolve over time. Sometimes, this is influenced by practitioners' professional explanations, sometimes from shared stories from other voice hearers, sometimes spiritual or religious influences might inform how voice hearing is understood, and many other sources can influence our beliefs. People can interpret and develop all sorts of beliefs about voice hearing experiences. Some may share similar ideas, but many will have different interpretations about voice hearing, and some of these interpretations may hold more weight and be privileged over other interpretations. Consequently, we believe it is important to remain open to learning and respecting different interpretations and associated meanings regarding voice hearing. Aligned with our beliefs about voice hearing, it was assumed throughout the research that no single "truth" or "reality" is out there waiting to be discovered or revealed through the analysis regarding voice hearing. Instead, ideas and assumptions about voice hearing are constructed, or developed, through a range of different sources of information and, from this, an understanding and associated meaning is developed, all of which isn't necessarily fixed but can change over time. The approach taken during the collection and analysis of information throughout the study similarly aligned with this interpretivist position, i.e., the development of the theory was shaped by the meaning co-developed jointly by both the people participating in the study (voice hearers and practitioners) and RA to provide an interpretation of voice-related experiences.

Having briefly outlined the research approach taken to develop the Tripartite Relationship Theory, we will now go on to examine in more detail in the next chapter the findings from talking to people about their voice hearing experiences.

Chapter 3

Hearing the "Personal Bully"

Voice hearing experiences

In the introduction to Part 2, we discussed the Grounded Theory research method-ology used to investigate voice hearing experiences, culminating in the develop-ment of the Tripartite Relationship Theory. In this chapter, we will consider the first of the two stages of the study, which involved talking to people about their voice hearing experiences. For this first stage, the aim was to understand how people in receipt of mental healthcare experienced voice hearing during their interactions with practitioners. Most of the participants used the term "patient" to describe their relationship with mental healthcare at the time of the study. We use this term here to reflect this and to align with the conventional use of it in the literature. How-ever, it is also important to note that not all participants were in receipt of mental healthcare at the time of the study and not all people who hear voices are in receipt of formal mental healthcare. We recognise this is a contested term and not appro-priate for everyone but is used here sparingly to differentiate people in receipt of healthcare from those providing healthcare. These interactions were between par-ticipants and practitioners and ranged from informal situations in healthcare such as everyday conversations to more formal procedures such as the administration of medication and care-related meetings. It involved any interaction with a practi-tioner and related to a healthcare experience during the person's time under the care of a mental health team. We begin by describing how participants were recruited for the study and how their experiences were collected and analysed.

Recruiting people to talk about their voice hearing experiences

The study took place in England, United Kingdom, and all but two people in this first stage of the study shared their experiences of receiving voice-related healthcare in a northern region of the country (the other two people had received care in the south). In the United Kingdom, most healthcare is provided by the National Health Service (NHS). Mostly, healthcare for those taking part in the study involved NHS Mental Health Services, comprising acute inpatient wards and community ser-vices such as Community Mental Health Teams, Assertive Outreach Teams and Early Interventions in Psychosis teams. To a lesser degree, healthcare in the United

DOI: 10.4324/9781032619910-5

Kingdom is also provided by private independent organisations, as was the case for some of the participants in the study. Such a broad range of clinical settings were included to help increase the opportunity to recruit people into the study.

Once in contact, Rob Allison (RA) asked participants if they could talk in a formally recorded semi-structured interview about their experiences of hearing voices during their times in mental healthcare settings and, specifically, during their interactions with healthcare practitioners. The interviews took place between October 2018 and October 2019. Of the 15 participants, there were seven males and eight females, aged between 18 and 63 years, and all had experienced mental healthcare settings (either inpatient or community). At the time of interview, several were in a mental healthcare setting, either community or residential-based; none were in a hospital setting at the time of interview. Eleven lived in their own home (either owned or rented), three lived in residential/supported accommodation, and one lived in a hostel. Five of the participants were in paid employment and one participated in voluntary work.

They all reported they heard voices and had received mental health treatment because of the distress they experienced in relation to their voices. We will return to the term treatment shortly to consider what this meant for people and their voices.

Power during interviews: people and voices

Taking part in an interview can reveal different levels of power, where an interviewer typically asks a range of questions to encourage the interviewee to disclose specific information. This can influence what is spoken by each and, for some interviewees, can be experienced as an abuse of power and, thus, requires the interviewer to be aware of how their own thoughts, feelings, and motivations might influence what they say or do during the interview (Aléx & Hammarström, 2008).

Typically, during an interview in this type of research study, the interviewee's shared experiences shape the conversation. Throughout the interviews in this study, all participants heard voices and most reported they actively heard voices throughout interview conversations. Interpersonal relationships can be experienced as traumatic and disempowering, both with other people and with voices, which can extend to relationships with practitioners (for example, see (Allison & Flemming, 2019). It was therefore important to avoid participants' feeling disempowered during interviews or feeling pressured to disclose information they might prefer to avoid.

Some participants reported their voices felt threatened during interviews and, in response, their voices sometimes became more aggressive. Some participants described physically feeling their voices moved closer towards them. For example, Diane, in her mid-50s and who lives with her son, described five regular and distressing voices, to which she linked past trauma. She explained that she had a difficult relationship with these voices, typically involving aggressive and hostile communication between Diane and the voices. Throughout the interview, Diane commented several times that either her voices were making aggressive and derogatory comments to her or she shouted (inside her head) profanities at the voices. Within the first couple of minutes of the interview, Diane commented "now they're [voices] just all jumping in, I can't understand anything now". Later in the interview, Diane described how one of her voices had reacted to a conversation during the interview and had moved around the room in response. Here is an excerpt from the conversation:

Interviewer: So, can you just describe that a bit more?
Diane: Sort of, like, when you're talking a bit intense, he thinks we're busy talking so he can just slip then and take whatever.
Interviewer: Okay, so in those conversations, does he come in closer?
Diane: Yes.
Interviewer: And how close would he get to you?
Diane: Kind of surrounding the top of us.
Interviewer: Okay, so he's all around you? [Diane nods]. All right, and then does he remain there all the time or does he move from there?
Diane: No, like, he can be above us or…
Interviewer: What happens when our conversation starts changing and we talk about other things, where does he go then?
Diane: Just sort of trying to get in any crack that he could in our conversation.
Interviewer: And with me being a male, what difference does it make to the position that he's in?
Diane: More fearful and respectful.
Interviewer: Okay. Do you know why that might be?
Diane: Because you're a man.
Interviewer: Do you think he worries about what I might do or…?
Diane: I think he knows that you're powerful.
Interviewer: And what does that do for you then if he's fearful and he's thinking I'm powerful?
Diane: Well, it's like I said to [CPN], if I got married, it would all disappear. If I had a big strong man, and he doesn't get us.
Interviewer: Okay. So does that mean then that if you were in a relationship with someone who was…
Diane: I think it [voices] would be different.

Diane's comments were not unusual for these interviews. Most participants reported that their voices commented on interview conversations. As another example, Clare had heard voices since her mid-teens (now in her mid-40s) and had received mental healthcare for around 20 years. She had lived alone for many years, heard numerous voices, which she described as a difficult relationship that typically caused her distress. She also reported her voices had commented to her at different points during the interview, making it difficult for her to hear: "they didn't like it earlier, when we were talking about authority". Later in the interview, Clare reported her voices were "telling me to fuck off or something…..it's got to do with [our discussion about] doctors and authority, I think". She attributed this to a power struggle with her voices, which was influenced by her own energy levels: "it's just my concentration", "[I don't] have the strength to fight them off". Earlier in the interview, Clare also disclosed that she had spent long periods of time in mental health inpatient units, detained under the Mental Health Act, at times escaped and subsequently returned by the police, and involuntary administered antipsychotic medication.

Sometimes during interviews, as we can see with Diane and Clare, voices became louder and generally more unpleasant (i.e., made derogatory comments and used foul language) towards participants, particularly when discussing difficult personal issues. This affected how participants responded to questions for fear of their voices' response. Consequently, when this happened, participants typically felt more distracted, anxious, or even distressed when the voices became more active. As such, it was important for RA to remain respectful and acknowledge their voices during interactions to help reduce some of the feelings of threat voices might experience, as reported by the participants. RA made a point of thanking the voices at the start and end of each interview and sometimes during the interviews and encouraged any voice-related distress to be openly acknowledged. A conversational style of interviewing developed, which was sensitive to increased voice activity, participants' distraction, their emotional state, and the importance of being attentive to the moment rather than following a script of questions. RA also regularly checked how participants felt and, when needed, short breaks were taken at various points during interviews.

Before we consider what participants said about their experiences of voice hearing and mental healthcare, we first explain in the section below the methods undertaken to analyse it.

Analysing what participants said during interviews

As we described in the introduction to Part 2, a number of key features or methods of Grounded Theory help to make it a distinct methodology and are required for the development of theory, which were utilised throughout this study. Analysis consisted of coding words or short phrases from transcriptions of the interviews that symbolised the interview data. Coding was a cyclical process that linked the interview data collection and the analysis of this data, which became increasingly conceptual to develop theory. Common to this methodology, there were three stages of coding, with several cycles of progressing through each stage: an initial open stage where codes were developed from the interview transcripts; a more advanced focused stage where categories of the initial codes were developed; and a theoretical stage where relationships between the categories were developed (Charmaz, 2014; Mills et al, 2006). Initial coding involved reading through the interview transcripts line by line and assigning names (codes) to relevant words or sections of transcripts that represented the meaning of what participants said. This gradually merged into the focused coding stage, which began to advance the theoretical direction of the analysis (Charmaz, 2014). This reflected the formation of categories of initial codes from the first stage and relationships between codes began to develop and move the analysis beyond a descriptive level. As the analysis of the interview data became increasingly conceptual, theoretical coding began. Increasingly conceptual categories of codes were developed eventually into six themes:

Personal bully
Biomedical treatment: limited involvement or fearing enforcement
Agency
Making sense of voices
Relating
Practitioners' actions

We will now explain each of the themes by sharing some of the experiences reported by the participants before we illustrate how they each relate with one another and form the initial development of the theory.

Personal bully

Participants heard voices before, during and after their contact with mental health services. Their experiences of their voices were influenced by their interactions with practitioners and the care they received during their time in services. They all reported they heard voices that were critical, abusive, insulting, and would taunt them. For example, their voices told them they deserved their previous abuse, and instructed them to hurt or kill themselves and/or other people. This, typically, contributed to a hostile relationship between participants and their voices. (It is important to note that not all voices were perceived in this way, but we will return to this shortly). The name of this theme comes from one of the participants, Noel, who described one of his voices as being his "own little personal bully". This term captured the way in which these types of voices were experienced. Ian had heard three voices until his dominant voices killed off one of his voices, which we will also come back to shortly to explain in more detail. During his interview, Ian reflected that his dominant voice would taunt him about previous abuse he had experienced:

> [Dominant voice] was laughing. I can remember it clearly. Yeah, he was laughing. He thought it was very funny and he was showing me the abuse…and that's the times when I was scared and distressed and acted on it and he said that I… you know, I should just kill myself, I shouldn't be here, and stuff like that.

During participants' interactions with other people, including practitioners, often their voices constantly talked and sometimes contradicted everything the participant said while they tried to hold a conversation. For example, during interactions with others, Noel's voices told him he was stupid and other people wouldn't believe him. Furthermore, and in addition to being taunted by their voices, participants were also discouraged by their voices from either helping themselves or reaching out to others to seek help. Kevin, for example, reported his voices called him a fool whenever he had tried to do something helpful for himself; similarly, Edith's voices did not like her attending appointments with practitioners and became louder; Noel's voices hated him going to therapy to receive help; and Clare's voices became louder whenever she tried to be kind to herself to cope with the distress from her voices. A consequence of these increased voice activities for participants was the increased difficulty for them to reach out for, and to receive, any support. This could, understandably, be perceived by others as avoiding or being dismissive of support.

The incessant nature of derogatory and interruptive voices, unsurprisingly, affected how participants perceived themselves and the intentions of others, including practitioners. This led to a difficult intra-inter-personal dynamic. For example, Hillary believed that because her voices had no respect for her, practitioners also did not respect her. As such, she had poor self-worth and perceived this was confirmed through her interactions with others. Another consequence of having constantly heard voices perceived as a personal bully was that participants became suspicious of practitioners' intentions. Bella's voices, for example, would tell her that practitioners intended to "section" her (meaning, she would be detained under the Mental Health Act).

Participants came to the attention of mental health services because of the distress related to their voice hearing. Most participants reported their voices to be mood-related: generally, the more stressed participants felt, the worse their voices became. Once admitted to services, they encountered practitioners and received healthcare largely underpinned by a biomedical approach. We turn to this healthcare approach in the next theme.

Biomedical treatment: limited involvement or fearing enforcement

All participants reported they had been prescribed psychotropic medication as a form of treatment to stop their voices and/or reduce their distress. This theme is two-fold in that it encapsulates participants' experiences of a biomedical response to voice-related distress through the widespread administration of psychotropic medication as "treatment"; and participants' fear that such so-called treatment would be administered involuntary, i.e., enforced.

Psychotropic medication was beneficial to some extent for some of the participants, for example Ian reported that it had previously helped to lift his mood; Liam, Edith, and Kevin reportedly found the blunting effect of medication on their emotions sometimes helped them feel less affected by their voices; and Hillary and Bella found the drowsiness effects of the medication could be helpful.

However, any benefit for participants was generally limited and did little to change the voices and underlying issues related to voice hearing. For example, Hillary also reflected she "realised that all of this medication was actually not stopping the issues" she had. Returning to Ian, when asked whether medication changed his voice hearing, he replied "no...I can honestly say that it didn't do nothing for me...[it] didn't stop the voices".

In fact, most participants reportedly felt worse because of psychotropic medication. For example, Bella gained three stone (21 kg) in weight, Ian slurred his words as a result of taking medication, Olivia found that she could hardly stand up or speak due to the medication, and Edith reported that her voices made it difficult for her to take medication: "Getting my tablets down is quite a struggle, because one of my voices doesn't like me having the tablets...But that, again, is like a power struggle within". The relationship participants had developed with medication was complex in so much as they reported mixed beneficial and deleterious effects from using it. For example, Frank described his medication as a "chemical cosh", but he also benefitted from the dampening down of his emotions.

Mostly, participants reported that the limited impact of medication on their voices and the side effects led them to believe they either didn't need to use medication or they wanted to reduce the dosage of their prescription. However, participants also reported they received insufficient support from practitioners to reduce or come off medication. As such, participants such as Liam took action into their own hands and immediately stopped taking it. Unsurprisingly, stopping medication abruptly in this way led to further distress for Liam (we were unable to confirm whether this was due to a drug withdrawal effect), and he soon recommenced medication. Similarly for Olivia, who also attempted to come off her medication and, when she found this difficult, she spoke with her psychiatrist who then re-prescribed her the medication.

Participants reported that medication was the only real treatment option they were provided, and it was administered through a range of coercive approaches by practitioners. Not only did the participants have a complex relationship with medication in terms of benefits and side effects, the decision-making about medication with practitioners was also opaque. During earlier stages in some interviews, some participants reported they had been involved by practitioners in decision-making regarding their treatment, specifically medication. However, they would also later report that their involvement in treatment-related decisions was actually quite limited, which was determined by the extent to which they agreed to accept medication. Olivia reflected on this: "I don't really get a choice, no, they just say, oh, this and this, I can choose if I want lemon or tutti-frutti in the calcium tablets". Liam reported that he had felt involved in treatment decisions when he reported that practitioners had asked him questions about establishing the right dosage of medication for him. He would later reflect, however, that he didn't know what his treatment comprised, and he took medication because he had been told to do so by his psychiatrist.

So, on the one hand, it could be argued that participants were involved in discussions with practitioners about decisions related to their own treatment, but this was limited to discussions that focused on *accepting* the treatment decision made by the practitioner. This, invariably, involved medication. This questions the extent to which participants were able to genuinely influence decisions made about their own treatment. When Clare became so frustrated with her lack of involvement in treatment decisions, she disengaged from mental health services only to find herself placed under further restrictions:

> I have been in services a long time. Yes, that would be to do with being told what I can and cannot do, I should imagine, it's pushed all the wrong buttons, and so I've gone AWOL from hospitals, and all sorts of stuff. Harmed myself in hospital, or whatever, I've ended up going in section, after section, after section. Free will, I suppose, it's freedom, free will, being free.

Most participants perceived an overarching force of mental healthcare and treatment, predominantly comprising psychotropic medication, which could be administered involuntarily, and which could be experienced as traumatic. Such an overarching coercive presence contributed to a fear of involuntary administration of psychotropics or the use of the Mental Health Act. Participants reported that practitioners strongly encouraged the use of psychotropic medication to treat their voice hearing. The underlying pressure applied by practitioners and perceived by participants was captured by Frank when he stated: "the only thing practitioners are good at is giving me medication". This highlighted a power imbalance between participants and practitioners. For example, Kevin reflected on a time when he had been distressed by his voices and he received a visit from a clinical team:

> Practitioners were literally sat there for like 10–20 minutes looking at me, saying 'take the drugs'. And I was like no, and it got to the point where I was just sat there not saying a word and these two doctors were sat on the sofa just looking at me saying, 'take them'. And it got to the point where no one was speaking. They were just sat there staring at me.

The first two themes we have described so far, "Personal Bully" and "Biomedical Treatment", represent a context in which voice hearing is experienced longer term. In other words, all participants heard voices they reported as distressing, which led to their admission into mental health services and in which they received predominantly medication as a "treatment" for their voice-related distress.

It is within this mental healthcare context that the next four themes are situated.

Agency

Hillary was in her mid-40s at the time of interview and had been in receipt of mental health services for the past 20 years. She lives with her partner in their own private accommodation and works in full-time employment. Hillary hears five voices, to which she attributes trauma she experienced earlier in her life. Over the years, she learned to relate to her voices by giving time regularly to listen to them, which she found reduced the power she believed they held over her. For Hillary, "voice hearing is about power and control". "Agency" represents this power in terms of the influence participants perceived they had regarding their voices and their subsequent "treatment".

Mostly, participants believed they had little to no agency over their voices. Typically, they felt overpowered by them. Interestingly, this also extended to relationships between different voices. Several participants (such as Alan, Ian, Edith and Mike) talked about difficulties between different voices, which involved power struggles between voices: some voices were dominant, some neutral or even friendly, and some were protective of the voice hearing participant and stood up against dominant abusive voices. For example, Ian, aged 48 years at the time of interview, had heard voices for the previous four years, to which he attributed trauma related to previous abuse he had experienced. Initially he heard three voices, but this was reduced to two when his dominant voice killed one of his other voices, as he described: "I only had [a male voice] for probably a month or two and then [the dominant voice] hurt him and showed me like images of him dead". The dominant voice would then show Ian images of the dead voice and would carry the head of the dead voices "around his belt…around his waist he'd got a belt with hooks on and he had (the dead voice's) head on a hook and he used to show me that all the time". Ian believed this act of violence by one voice onto another voice was about demonstrating to him "power to make me scared so that I would listen to him".

Participants perceived their voices were constantly attempting to gain an upper hand, to be in control over the participant in some way. Sometimes, the wrestling between participants and their voices would become increasingly hostile and participants would reciprocate with abusive language to their voices. We touched on this a little earlier in the chapter with Diane when she reported that she had shouted back and swore (in her head) to her voices during our interview.

Several participants explained how they engaged in self-injurious behaviours because of their distress attributed to their voices. Edith was in her 30s at the time of interview, had heard voices for 17 years, and lived with her partner and engaged in voluntary work. She heard three individual voices and also a crowd of voices and, consistent with other participants, attributed them to previous traumatic experiences. Edith felt overwhelmed by her voices to the extent that sometimes she would self-injure as a way of creating some peace with them. Her comments reveal a battle of attrition:

> They have always had a hold on me…the things that they've made me do…they would go at me and go at me…to the point where I couldn't take it anymore. And then it would be too much. And then something would happen…it was that kind of power that they would have.

Later in the interview, Edith commented:

> It was very much kind of a double thing with the hurting myself, because I would hurt myself to do as they said, but also when I hurt myself, they would go away because they got what they wanted. So it would yeah. It would just be so much easier to hurt myself and have that peace.

To counter this, most participants attempted to empower themselves in relation to their voices. They did this by participating in a range of activities as an attempt to either directly or indirectly increase their perceived agency over their voices and reduce distress related to them. We can see this with examples from Kevin, Bella, Glenda, Jenny, Hillary, Mike, Clare, Diane, Ian, and Frank, who all utilised different ways to empower themselves. Kevin, a 23-year-old who lived in a residential house, had only heard voices for one year at the time of interview. He volunteered at his local RSPCA as a way of helping animals and people, which enabled him to put his voices aside at least temporarily. Bella had heard voices for approximately 20 years from her early teenage years. In her 40s at the time of interview, she heard three voices and, in contrast to some of the other participants, we have introduced so far, Bella attempted to keep a distant relationship with her voices, which also reflected her relationship with other people. Bella found that playing musical instruments helped to intercept her voices, providing her with evidence that she was able to influence her voices at times. Glenda, a 63-year-old who heard one voice, and Jenny, also in her 60s and who heard three voices, and Hillary, who we met earlier, all found employment to be a helpful way of shifting their focus away from their voices, thus reducing the extent to which their voices dominated their daily lives. Jenny, additionally, found activities such as writing poetry or practising mindfulness techniques helpful. Mike, a 20-year-old who had heard several voices for three years, found researching into his voices contributed to him believing them to be a spiritual awakening and over which he had power and control. Clare, whom we met earlier in the chapter, found yoga and conscious efforts to ground herself physically to things such as the pavement were useful approaches. Diane, whom we also met earlier, found reaching out and asking for help and attending a local Hearing Voices group helped her gain some influence over her voices and reduce some of the power she believed they previously had over her. These activities were not completely successful per se at stopping the voices from causing distress but the action of doing something, of engaging in something meaningful for the individual, helped to improve the experience of voice hearing, albeit temporary.

Regarding influencing the power participants perceived their voices held over them, three particularly interesting methods stood out. The first involved disclosure of voices. All participants kept their voices private and, upon first hearing them, concealed them from others. At some point later in their voice hearing experiences, they all also eventually disclosed their voices to others. This action of disclosure was a seemingly effective way of empowering oneself in relation to the voices. This was most explicitly described by Diane, who was regularly taunted by voices about her childhood abuse, when she talked about the shame and power related to voice hearing:

> After you've been abused, you spend your life trying to be normal anyway, and you feel contagious. But [the voices] latched onto that kind of thing because it was a secret, they could do all that in my head...[and later]...When they're a secret in your head, they [voices] have a lot more power, you know, like I would

hurt myself. I would just sit all day…it [one of the voices] was just telling us how…the reasons things happened to us, because I deserved it.

Diane went on to explain the power of disclosure:

Because I was saying to the voices 'I'm not keeping any more secrets', this is the beginning, 'you start torturing us again and I'm going to speak up about it', it seemed for a little while anyway they backed off, and it wasn't constant 'you're useless', you know, 'go kill yourself', 'go and do this', and I got out a bit, you know? Out to meet friends and that, and going for a coffee, whereas before when I was just stuck there, I couldn't…the voices were too powerful, I couldn't answer the phone never mind meet someone for a cup of coffee.

The second method related to whether voices were acknowledged or ignored. Participants reported their voices did not like being ignored; voices wanted to be heard and acknowledged. Those who ignored their voices reported they perceived they had little to no influence regarding the extent to which voices were interruptive and, consequently, distressing. However, participants such as Diane, Edith, Hillary, and Noel recognised that ignoring them made their voices stronger, louder and angrier and so they made sure to set aside time regularly to listen to their voices. This contributed to developing some agency over their voices in terms of reducing the intensity of the voice hearing experiences. Perhaps, the most fascinating account of spending planned time with voices came from Frank. He had constructed an imaginary garden in his mind, which comprised beautiful greenery, trees, and a bridge by a stream in what Frank described as a serene place:

When I want to talk to my voices, I go to the garden myself and I talk to my voices in the garden and I found that I have a much better conversation with them there, because they're not out and seeing everything and being scared and they're in this nice relaxing place with a nice pool and trees and tree house and all sorts of nice things there, nice little stream.

Described in this way we can see, through constructing this process of engaging with his voices, Frank developed some agency and, consequently, ability to assert some control over his voices.

The third method involved taking responsibility for one's actions. We can see this in several ways with Hillary, Clare, Frank, and Jenny. For example, Hillary took responsibility for setting time limits with her voices to contain some of the impact of her voices on other areas of her life and, overall, to manage her voices. She stated: "I have to set boundaries for myself. Not just with [voices], but in my life, I've found that I've had to do that. I've had to change my whole life, because of [voices]".

Taking responsibility took a different form for Clare. Instead, for her, this concerned owning her own contribution to distress. Clare decided she no longer wanted to use alcohol and cannabis instead wanted a cleaner life to help her manage her voices.

Frank similarly wanted to accept responsibility for his own actions, which followed a time when his voices told him to attack a stranger whilst walking in the park one day. He found the garden he had created in his mind, mentioned earlier in the chapter, helped him to calm his voices and Frank began to learn how to manage future commands from his voices. Finally, taking responsibility for Jenny involved accepting her voices as her own: "Nobody else can hear these, these are mine. These are mine and I'm ready to own them…now I will take ownership and say, right, this is my issue". This led to her becoming interested in understanding where the voices came from: "they're my voices, therefore it's up to me to find out what's going on for me".

Making sense of voices

Participants constructed personal meaning of some sort regarding their voice hearing, which involved a long-term process of making sense of their voices prior to, during and following admission to mental health services. From the early stages of voice hearing, participants began to learn about their voices either through self-discovery, such as reading about voice hearing and/or engaging with their voices, and/or through engaging with others (this would typically be practitioners when in mental health services or other voice hearers). "Making sense of voices" represents this process.

The participants were all at different stages of making their own sense of their voice hearing. For those who had heard voices longer term, they reported their sense-making had changed over time. Most had also learned somehow to tolerate their voices. Exceptions to this were those such as Kevin, who had heard voices for a comparatively shorter time (under two years) and had yet to make sense of who/what his voices were or even why he heard voices. Consequently, Kevin had not found an effective way of relating or managing his voices and even found it difficult to differentiate himself from his voices:

> "Sometimes it's one person and they'll say, "it's only me". But then I get other voices saying "no, it's me as well"… there's loads, like there's multiple people in my head, like well multiple voices. So I don't know if it's one person trying other voices on…[and later]…I don't know if it's my fault or my voices putting ideas into my head…I don't know if it's my decision or my voices saying go and do this".

Mike had heard voices for a little longer than Kevin (for three years) but, through actively researching and reading about voice hearing, he changed his initial understanding of voices and came to believe that his voices were a guide to help him appreciate a better perspective of life and to learn how to "deal with things". Glenda believed her voices were external to herself and were aliens. Most, however, identified their voices as part of themselves. For example, Bella believed her voices were the paranoid and critical parts of herself, and Noel believed one of his voices was his early teen self who was quiet and had "shut down from the world". We touched on a fascinating account by Frank in the previous "Agency" theme. Frank, you may remember, had created an imaginary garden in his mind where he would take his voices. He had spent a lot of time reading about voice hearing and reflecting on his own experiences to help him understand how his voice hearing was linked to previous childhood trauma. This led to him believing that his voices are:

> different parts of myself, like split off parts of my personality, basically whenever I've had a tragedy in my life, my personality has split off at that point and it's become a voice…[and later]….the five year old told me that it was a child and I worked out myself it was, because of the way it acted, it was the same way as I used to act when I was that age and that's, sort of, gave me the indication that the rest of them were part of my personality as well.

Making sense was an important process to begin and engage with for participants to improve their voice hearing experience. Extending this, being able to identify voices as part of oneself was also important in terms of accepting voice hearing, accepting oneself, and relating more positively with voices. Most participants associated their voice hearing with an earlier traumatic event(s) of some sort. Returning to Frank, he benefitted from identifying his voices as part of himself and rooted in earlier childhood trauma. He believed making this link helped him to relate with himself and his voices:

> It showed me first of all that I was worth loving, which meant that the voices must be worth loving too, because they were part of me. So, I sort of, started to try and see them in a different way and try and give them love. Especially the five-year-old, I mean, the 10-year-old, seven-year-old and the 14-year-old are not really interested, you know, but the five-year-old really craves it. So, yeah, it helped a lot.

In addition to hearing a voice, most participants reported they saw a presence (visual image) they associated with a voice. All associated the images of their voices with previous trauma. They also reported their images to be mobile so they moved to different areas in a room, for example, and moved closer or further away from the participant. We introduced you to Ian earlier in the chapter and described his experience of initially hearing three voices, which reduced to two when his dominant voice killed one of his other voices. Ian had a very traumatic experience during his childhood, when he was sexually abused by a local vicar. Later, in adulthood, he began to hear voices, one of which was perceived as the most dominant voice and was always accompanied by a clear image of a reverend, dressed in a long black cloak and hood, and would move around:

> when I've been driving the van I seen him in the passenger seat. I see him sometimes when I'm sat on the couch [at home]. He can be the other side of the room. If I'm down the farm he could be in the field.

For Olivia, voice hearing mostly involved only an audio experience, i.e., she heard her voices but did not experience any other sensation associated with her voices. However, during more stressful periods, she also experienced a visual image of her voices, which she reported could vary between her different voices. Olivia became more anxious with the presence of a visual image as she associated this with her voices becoming increasingly powerful and her lack of ability to contain them in her head. One of the participants, Alan, didn't see a visual image of his voices but, instead, he sensed a physical presence he associated with his dominant voice. He located this image on the other side of a wall of any room he entered so that it always remained present but out of sight.

Relating

This concerns how participants related both with their voices and with practitioners. Participants had mixed experiences of relating: some had positive relationships with some of their voices but difficult relationships with other voices; similarly, they reported examples of positive experiences with practitioners, but they had also experienced difficulties during their interactions and relationships with some practitioners.

Interestingly, the relationship participants had developed with their voices mirrored, to some extent, their relationships with other people. Noel, for example, would respond to increased hostility from his dominant voice by barricading himself in his room to hide from the voice; he would similarly hide away from other people at times of distress. Clare also reported that she tended to run away from difficult situations at various points in her life just as she tried to run away from her voices and keep a distance from distressing situations. Frank, on the other hand, had learnt to look after his voices (you may remember, he takes them to his imaginary garden) and he also reported that he liked to look after his wife by cooking her meals and buying her flowers. The following quote from Bella encapsulates the mirroring of relating with voices and people: "my own kind of anxious avoidant pattern of relating, is manifested in the way that I've learned to relate to the voices".

Participants generally found it difficult to talk to others about their voice hearing and related problems. An important factor contributing to this was participants' concerns regarding whether people would believe them. Alan, for example, stopped going to therapy to avoid talking about his voices; Edith was fearful of talking about her voices because she usually experienced a backlash from them; Bella found it difficult to talk about her past abuse for fear of not being believed or being perceived as delusional. Ian also feared not being believed. He concealed his childhood abuse for years:

> I couldn't even tell my mum and dad because I was scared of not being believed because, you know, somebody in the church, you know, he was like in a good standing in the community, and that. So, I was just scared of not being believed.

Participants reported that feeling accepted as a voice hearer and supported was important to improving their experience of hearing voices. Almost exclusively, this feeling of acceptance and support came from socialising with other people who similarly heard voices and experienced difficulties related to this. Hearing Voices Groups were identified by several participants as especially supportive but also family, friends, and peers.

Practitioners were also considered by participants as supportive, not always but at various points during times spent in mental health services. This was categorised into two groups: participants providing general interactions and participants engaging more directly with voice hearing. Regarding the first group, participants reported their general interactions with practitioners were supportive. For example, Kevin found it helpful when he was in an inpatient ward and a practitioner would talk to him about general issues; Liam and Noel both valued times when practitioners demonstrated care towards them; Frank and Clare both valued practitioners who supported them to problem solve; Bella appreciated practitioners who listened to her rather than medicalise her struggles; when Olivia and Hillary became distressed they could sometimes feel contained by practitioners, an example of which is provided by which Hillary when she reflected on her time in an inpatient unit:

> She came down and sat on the floor with me. So, she came down to the level I was at, and talked to me until I felt able that I could uncurl myself and sit back in a chair. She didn't threaten me, she didn't tell me to stop being stupid. She realised I was in distress, and that was my safety, my position of safety, because of the battering I was taking from the voices, I just wanted to curl up in a ball, because I didn't want to be there. I didn't want to be alive, but I didn't want to end it, so the safety position was to curl up in a ball. And she came down and sat on the floor and talked to me like a human being. And gave me that time, until I could uncurl myself, and with her help, get sat back on the bed. And I realised, then, that she probably did actually care.

The second group concerned practitioners who focused more directly on specifically four participants' (Jenny, Mike, Ian, and Hillary) voice hearing experiences. For example, returning to Hillary, she found it helpful when a particular practitioner she recalled had encouraged her to accept she heard voices and offered her advice to help her manage her voice hearing when in public situations. Jenny, Mike, and Ian had all engaged in talking therapy, which involved focusing specifically on their voice hearing. Ian reflected: "from the start of the therapy things just started to get a little bit better with me understanding the voices, how they're associated, and how I control them now".

Interestingly, Jenny, Mike, Ian, and Hillary all developed relatively higher perceived levels of agency in their relationships with their voices and other people. All four had developed a way of relating they found effective with their voices, a way to manage voice-related distress, and/or they had gained employment and managed relationships with others.

Trust was a particularly important factor for participants, both inter-personally with others and intra-personally with voices. It was difficult for participants to feel they could trust others, but it was an important factor in feeling supported by practitioners. It took participants' time to feel able to trust other people, practitioners included, and typically, this was made more challenging due to the comments made by their voices. Voices often told participants not to trust practitioners or others, but participants also struggled to relate with and trust their voices. Having heard of the benefit of improving and developing positive relationships with voices from other people who heard voices, Clare tried but struggled:

> It was once mentioned that if I give them some love and attention, caring changes the whole relationship with them, it might help. It's just something I can't do with them. And, with some of the voices being so close, they're actually with me most of the time, I don't know how to love them, or give them that care and attention that they probably need.

Most participants at some point attempted to conceal their voice hearing due to their fear of receiving a diagnosis of schizophrenia and of receiving threats from their voices. As such, some had been able to conceal their voice hearing from practitioners. For example, Diane spent one year in a therapeutic community but had been able to conceal her voices from her peers and practitioners.

Some participants, such as Liam, Noel, Bella, Diane, and Glenda, reported they wanted to get rid of their voices, or if not all their voices, then at least the dominant abusive ones. One of the ways participants tried to manage their difficult relationships with voices was to distance themselves from their voices. For example, Bella consciously developed an emotionally distant relationship with her voices, which she termed "minimal relating":

> I'd worked on not having a relationship with the.... to not have a relationship with something that you hear, is quite a complicated thing. But what I mean by that is that I choose to kind of have distance from it, and before it says something, just either in my head, question it, or dismiss it. Not kind of have any emotional connection with it.

Although Bella utilised distancing and emotional disconnection from her voices, distancing oneself from voices also led to other participants ignoring, or attempting to ignore, their voices, which made them worse. You may remember when we discussed the "Agency" theme that participants also said their voices wanted to be acknowledged. As such, attempts to ignore voices were typically fraught with conflict. For example, Jenny reported that the more tried to push her voices away, the more they would push back at her:

> They would go at me, they were horrible to me, and I didn't want them anymore. And I would try not to engage with them, because I just think that would have

encouraged them. I don't know if I'm right or wrong, I don't know because I've never tried it, I didn't want to.

We stated in the "Personal Bully" theme that not all voices were hostile nor all voice hearer-voice relationships abusive or distressing. Participants described a complex set of relationships with voices, wherein they experienced distressing relationships with some voices but positive relationships with other voices. In other words, voice hearing per se was not problematic for participants. Rather, the relationship they had with their voices determined whether their experience of voice hearing was problematic. For example, Kevin liked to have his voices with him when he was sat alone doing nothing; Diane reported she would be lonely without her voices; Ian, Mike, Liam, and Noel all described good relationships with some of their voices; indeed, Noel's voices encouraged him to go to therapy and Mike reported his voices were like a teacher or guide to him.

In contrast to Bella's "minimal relating" approach, Hillary, Frank, and Jenny changed their distressing voice hearing experiences they previously had by making a conscious decision to change how they related to their voices. We have already heard about some of Hillary's and Frank's experiences and so let us close the discussion on this code with a quote from Jenny. Jenny learnt that her voices served an important function in suppressing her emotions, which enabled her to function in life to some extent. As such, she reflected on the purpose of relating positively with her voices:

> You can only do that for so long, I think. I tried to keep the voices at a distance, I tried to ignore, but they have an impact on all of your life. So, if you're gonna try and get on with your life...I always remember saying to one doctor, I just want my life back. Maybe not to how it was, but I needed some sort of life. And if that means that I try to have a relationship with my voices, then so be it.

Practitioners' actions

This final theme represents participants' perceptions regarding practitioner involvement in their voice hearing experiences during their time in mental health services. Their reported experiences illustrate the important role and subsequent effect of the way in which they experience their voices. Previously in the "Relating" theme, we discussed how participants valued the support offered by practitioners, both in terms of their general approach and one that specifically focused on voice hearing. However, overall, participants mostly reported that practitioners failed to demonstrate sufficient understanding of their difficulties, generally, and voice hearing specifically.

Participants reported that, generally, they perceived that practitioners failed to fully appreciate their experiences of voice hearing. They reported that practitioners' suggested coping strategies such as walking or taking hot baths were usually unhelpful and insensitive. Mike, reported that practitioners were more concerned with monitoring his level of risk than they were with understanding his voice-related difficulties; Diane and Clare believed practitioners didn't genuinely listen to them and, consequently, they felt unable to talk with practitioners; Bella and Glenda believed practitioners had lacked genuine hope for their recovery; indeed, Bella reported that practitioners told her to lower her expectations of life and Glenda believed practitioners had encouraged her to give up her employment due to stress when in fact she believed her stress was related to her voices rather than employment; and the following quotes from Edith illustrate a lack of therapeutic quality in her perception of her interactions with practitioners:

> "Some of their attitudes, they're just like that they don't want to help, that they're just there for the money and just weren't very engaging, and just kind of sat there and didn't do things". [And later…] "But some of the healthcare assistants would just sit there and chat to each other, and wouldn't do anything with you… and when you're just sat there all day with nothing to do but sit and listen to your voices, it's not very helpful". [And later…] "All we did all day was just sit and watch the telly. And that's why you'd end up trying to find ways to hurt yourself, just to get that peace. And it's not easy to hurt yourself on a secure unit. But that's what you did because all you wanted to do was get that peace in your head, so you would try and hurt yourself because that's just…it was very, very, what's the word – intense, very intense".

More specifically, participants reported that practitioners failed to talk with them in any meaningful way about their voice hearing. Diane, Kevin, Liam, Alan, Edith, Frank, Noel, Jenny, and Olivia all reported a lack of discussion with practitioners about their voice hearing. At best, any discussion involved practitioners simply checking if their voices were better or worse than previously. Diane believed practitioners invalidated her voice hearing and felt uncomfortable talking to her about voices, instead signposting her to a Hearing Voices Group:

Diane:	Because it makes people uncomfortable and practitioners, it makes them uncomfortable as well.
Interviewer:	What makes them uncomfortable?
Diane:	Hearing voices…because they don't know…
Interviewer:	So you think practitioners find it uncomfortable when talking about voices? What do you think it is then that makes them uncomfortable?
Diane:	Because they can't just give you a pill.

Another way in which practitioners were perceived as being unhelpful to participants was their pathologising of voice hearing and interpretation of it as a symptom of a mental disorder. Some participants, such as Jenny and Olivia, were given more than one diagnosis, namely, schizophrenia and borderline personality disorder. Bella, Liam, Jenny, Mike, and Olivia all reported their voice hearing had been framed with a diagnosis of schizophrenia. Bella's fear of this diagnosis led her to conceal her voices for several years. She reported she had attended an appointment with a psychiatrist on one occasion and inadvertently discovered she had been diagnosed with schizophrenia when the psychiatrist left the room momentarily but had left Bella's medical notes open for her to see. Mike also had a similar experience of passively discovering his diagnosis of schizophrenia:

> Well, when they told me the diagnosis they did it like the guy said it like so slyly, like he just like slipped it in there....he was like, do you know you're paranoid schizophrenic? And I was like, I just went, yeah, I do, but like I was a bit, yeah.

Generally, participants believed that rather than develop personally meaningful discussion about voice hearing, practitioners attempted to fit their voice hearing experiences and related difficulties into a professional framework, such as diagnostic categories or Cognitive Behavioural Therapy or recovery models.

Summary of themes

Overall, from analysing the information gleaned from the interviews, we can make sense of the participants' experiences according to how they relate to their voices and practitioners, their level of distress associated with their voices, and their perceived level of agency. Figure 3.1 illustrates the integration of the six inter-related themes to encapsulate the participants' voice hearing experiences during their interactions with practitioners and within a mental healthcare context.

We can see from this that six participants (Frank, Hillary, Ian, Jenny, Mike, and Noel) generally have more comparatively positive relationships with their voices, more perceived agency regarding their voices and treatment, are comparatively less distressed by their voices, and value their voices to some extent. By contrast, the other nine participants (Alan, Bella, Clare, Diane, Edith, Glenda, Kevin, Liam, and Olivia) relate negatively with their voices, lack agency with their voices and treatment, are comparatively more distressed from hostile and critical voices, and want to get rid of their voices.

Theoretical explanation of participants' experiences

The analysis led to an initial theoretical explanation of the experiences of people who hear voices within a mental healthcare context. Further research and subsequent analysis helped to develop this further into the Tripartite Relationship Theory, more of which we discuss in the next two chapters. At this point specifically concerning voice hearer experiences, however, we propose that a largely biomedical treatment context and inter-personal relations shape intra-personal experiences of voice hearing.

People who hear voices and receive mental healthcare will have heard voices before their first contact with mental health services and, thus, their first interaction

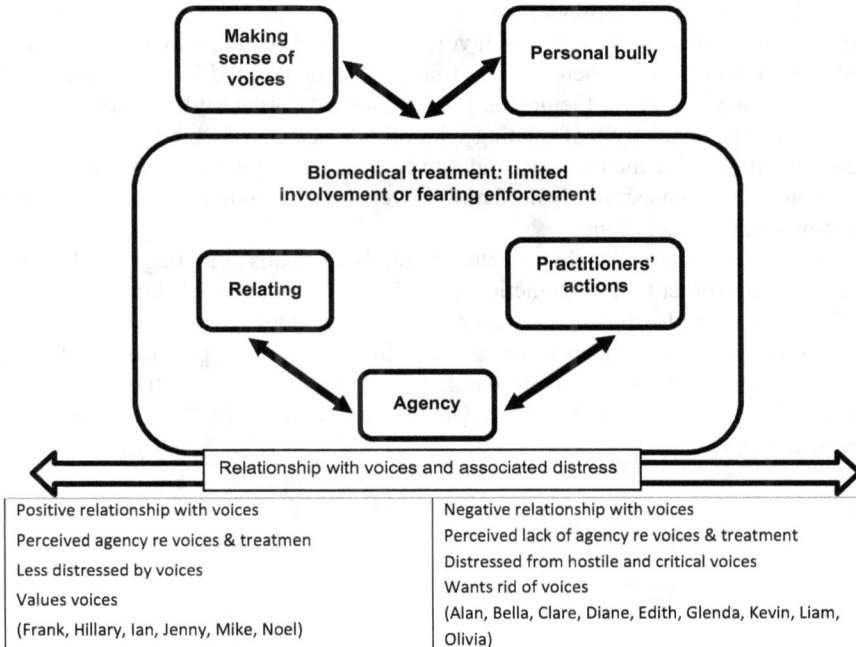

Figure 3.1 Inter-related themes for voice hearers.

with a practitioner. Following their first voice hearing experience, they will have already begun to develop thoughts about their voices and, to varying degrees, begun to try to make sense of what is happening to them. This sense-making typically evolves over time and possibly becomes a life-long journey. For those who eventually come into contact with mental health services, they experience their voices as hostile, abusive, and overpowering, akin to a Personal Bully. For this group of people, both their efforts to make sense of their voices and their experience of voice hearing develop both outside of their time spent in mental health services and during it. Once admitted into mental health services, people hearing voices typically perceive healthcare to lack any real genuine choice of support, with medication conventionally administered as "treatment" for their voice hearing and voice-related distress. Mostly, voice hearers believe they are expected by practitioners to accept medication and, should they refuse, they fear they will be coerced by practitioners into complying.

Extending this, these experiences involve the use of power, specifically coercion. We can see that power is present in the nature and content of voices. Indeed, the theme "Personal Bully" represents the overpowering effect of voices on the voice hearer. "Agency" also represents the level of influence, and thus power, voice hearers have over their voice hearing experience. When voices are interruptive, hostile, and abusive, and where the voice hearer is unable to influence this, it infers that the voice hearer lacks sufficient power and, indeed, is overpowered. Furthermore, power is present in the way in which voice hearers relate not just with their voices but with practitioners. Where a person might feel persecuted by their voices and relate submissively with them, this intra-personal relating style appears to mirror an inter-personal style of relating with others, particularly practitioners. Voice hearers can perceive their voices hold power over them and they can also perceive that practitioners can similarly hold power over them through their interactions and treatment-related decisions.

As we have discussed in this chapter, the study up to this point began to illustrate a voice hearer-practitioner interaction, but with the intra-personal element in which the voice hearer also heard and experienced voices. One of the themes ("Practitioners' actions") concerns practitioners but this was from the perspective of voice hearing participants. To complete the development of the theory, the experiences of practitioners also needed to be understood, and this is what we will explore in the next chapter.

Chapter 4

Experiences of supporting people distressed by voice hearing

In Chapter 3, we discussed the experiences of people who have been distressed by voice hearing, their "personal bully", and have been in receipt of mental healthcare. One of the themes included in these experiences concerned the actions of practitioners. Voice hearing participants reported practitioners generally lacked sufficient knowledge and understanding of their difficulties and their voice hearing experiences. To further develop the Tripartite Relationship Theory of voice hearing, this second stage of the study explored further perceptions concerning practitioners' actions. The aim was to understand practitioners' perspectives regarding voice hearing through listening to their experiences of supporting and interacting with voice hearers.

Collecting information from practitioners

Following on from the first stage of the study, further theoretical development was required. This involved collecting information relating to voice hearing experiences from the perspectives of practitioners. Practitioners from northern and southern regions of a local NHS Trust, collectively supporting inpatient and community services, agreed to discuss their experiences in focus groups. This helped to provide information concerning the team approach, culture and gain some insight into the group dynamics within the clinical environment.

Three focus groups comprised a total of 18 practitioners, all of whom worked in the NHS and who shared their experiences over a duration of approximately one hour and over a two-week period in October 2019. Practitioners were from either the same clinical team (focus group one was an inpatient unit, focus group two from a community team) or the same service (focus group three from a psychosis specialist team) and in total comprised nine mental health nurses (RMN), four associate practitioners/support workers, three occupational therapists, one clinical psychologist, and one family therapist. Of the 18 practitioners, 16 were female and two were male, all were White British, ranging in age from 20s to 60s (years), and were on an NHS Agenda for Change grade banding from 4 to 8b. Their number of years of working with people who hear voices ranged from 6 months to 47 years, with an average of 13 years.

DOI: 10.4324/9781032619910-6

Analysing practitioners' experiences

You may remember we described in Chapter 3 a method known as theoretical sampling, which essentially for theory development informs the researcher of the type and source required for their next set of data (or information) for theory development. So, for example, with regard to the interviews with voice hearers discussed in Chapter 3, following this process enabled different types of information to be collected by asking different types of questions of voice hearers as the number of interviews progressed. In other words, to build theory, information collected from the first few people to be interviewed helped to inform different questions for different information required from people in later interviews. By the end of the first stage of the study, this subsequently led to identifying practitioners from whom to collect a different source of information (in this second stage) for the purpose of enhancing theory development. Consequently, analysis of the practitioner's information involved developing coding. In Chapter 5, we will explain how we then merged the two sets of coding from the interviews discussed in the previous chapter and the focus groups discussed in this chapter to complete theory development. For the remainder of this chapter, though, we will discuss the analysis (or coding) of practitioners' experiences.

In terms of the research method of coding, the level of analysis of the practitioners' experiences evolved to stage 2: focused coding (you may remember, when applying this methodology, analysis involves three levels of increasingly abstract coding to develop theory: initial, focused, and theoretical). This led to the development of six focused codes, which would eventually be synthesised with the findings from the individual interviews (discussed in Chapter 5) to complete the development of the tripartite relationship theory. These are described below with examples of some of the information practitioners discussed from across the three focus groups.

Challenges related to coercive practice

Practitioners reported a complex relationship with the concept of coercion, which mainly concerned the administration of medication and the use of the Mental Health Act. They believed coercion, at times, was a necessity to enable "treatment" but they also found the administration of it, and coercive practice in general, challenging. For example, in terms of legislation, practitioners valued the Mental Health Act as a means of legally permitting coercive practice to administer what they considered to be "treatment". One of the practitioners from the first focus group, Carrie, a mental health nurse, commented on this: "If someone is very, very distressed by voices, it's kind of heartbreaking, isn't it? You want to intervene. It seems cruel not to do something. And so, if the Mental Health Act didn't exist, would there be something else in place"?

Practitioners spoke about the negative consequences of coercion on voice hearing experiences. For example, although there were examples where application of the MHA was valued by practitioners, conversely some also believed that the MHA involved coercive practice such as the use of Community Treatment Orders. This enabled practitioners to recall patients to the hospital for failing to comply with medication, for example, which they believed typically strengthened patients' beliefs regarding the warnings of threat they heard from their voices. Practitioners also believed coercive practice such as this undermined the potential to create therapeutic relationships with patients, leading to "synthetic" rather than collaborative and trusting relationships. Discussion relating to this in the second focus group between three practitioners (Lucy and Jack, both mental health nurses, and Ken, a support worker) illustrates their frustration:

Lucy:	But also you've got the CTOs [Community Treatment Orders] and that. The amount of people who are on CTOs who hear voices…that's another massive barrier.
Ken:	They're not openly accessing our service, are they? They're not engaging with you because…
Jack:	That's power.
Ken:	…they want to. There's that power, isn't there?
Jack:	It's just total power, isn't it?

Practitioners, generally, spoke about feeling "horribly conflicted" regarding coercion. We get a flavour of this when we return to Carrie from the first focus group, who commented: "I suppose you're damned if you do [coerce] and damned if you don't. Sometimes it feels like you're stuck between a rock and a hard place". Consequently, practitioners sometimes found it difficult to uphold their professional accountabilities while simultaneously respecting patients' individual autonomy.

Interestingly, practitioners shared different ways they tried to soften the impact of coercion of patients. For example, practitioners from an acute ward in the first focus group believed they were helping patients work towards recovery by persuading them to engage in various occupational therapy activities on the ward, with an implicit understanding that patients' failure to attend would be construed as a failure to engage in treatment. Returning to the earlier point regarding the negative impact of coercion on relationships, practitioners talked about how they tried to protect the relationships certain members of the clinical team had with patients by removing those colleagues who had established positive relationships with a patient from coercive situations.

Regarding the feelings of conflict previously mentioned in relation to coercion, it was important for practitioners to be able to justify their coercive practice. Some said they believed that patients improved because of coercive interventions. To help justify coercively medicating patients, it was helpful for practitioners to believe there were longer term benefits of taking medication for patients. This also included situations when practitioners believed it was in a patient's best interests for practitioners to administer medication even when the patient begged not to have it. Some practitioners felt conflicted, though, in situations involving medication. For example, Ken from the second focus group recognised this as particularly concerning where a patient had a history of abuse:

> I think [we need] reviews of medication on where it's administered, you know, we work with a lot of people, experience sexual abuse, depot medication, usually in the rear. I don't think that's ever considered that much.

Practitioners talked about the importance of being honest and transparent with patients, especially when they anticipated coercive practice. Some practitioners from focus groups one and two reflected that they would discuss with patients their preferred injection sites should they need to be administered an injection of medication at a later date against their wishes. Practitioners from focus group three believed it was important for them to stay with patients during an act of coercion, for example application of the Mental Health Act to detain the patient, and to try to comfort the patient (i.e., with a cup of tea) whilst simultaneously trying to arrange an assessment to detain them under the Mental Health Act. This again reflects the complexity and conflict for practitioners.

A particularly interesting issue that became evident during focus group discussions concerned practitioners' understanding of what coercion is. For example, some practitioners were unable to differentiate between coercion and choice. For those patients who refused to take medication, practitioners were unsure whether their action of telling patients they could either accept oral medication or receive an enforced injection of medication was offering choice or being coercive. In another example, Sarah, an Occupational Therapist from the third focus group, reflected on her planned visit to a patient's home for the purpose of ensuring the patient remained compliant with their medication and remained in contact with the clinical team. It might be argued that Sarah did no more than try to gently persuade the patient to keep taking their medication and to keep in touch with the team, which might not be considered coercive. However, this interaction ought to be contextualised within a broader clinical approach in which the gentler, subtler approach is to persuade and, failing that, it is explicitly known by the patient and the team that a threat of harder forms of coercion (e.g., detainment under the Mental Health Act, enforced medication, etc.) can be utilised should the initial approaches fail. Patients' experiences of coercion ought to be considered within this broader context rather than isolated approaches. Arguably, this is problematic for practitioners in terms of defining and understanding coercion and the Mental Health Act can influence their perceptions about coercion and infer they are providing choice. Anne, an Associate Practitioner in focus group one, stated: "I think without the Mental Health Act you would absolutely think it's coercion. But because that's there it's almost...it's giving people some choice within...a lack of choice".

Extending this discussion further regarding the difficulty practitioners experienced with defining coercion, some practitioners normalised coercion and considered it an everyday phenomenon that happens between people. Take, for example, the discussion between Rose and Oriette, two mental health nurses in the third focus group:

Rose: I think coercion is a two-way street. I think we are coerced by our staff and peers into doing stuff that we haven't got the time to do it. And we do coerce our patients; it's not documented how we got Joe Blogs and [how] we coerced him. It's [documented] as gentle persuasion or encouragement or whatever. It's the transparent tool that sometimes has to be used, mainly the path of least resistance. [Agreement in the group] That's what it is. We do it with kids and everything.

Oriette: And it's about the best interest of the patient, isn't it?

Rose: Of course it is. And we do it with kids.

Understanding the concept of coercion and administering coercive practice can be complex and challenging for practitioners. Some struggled to recognise coercion and sometimes reframed it as giving choice to patients or underplayed the powerful and negative effects of it by normalising it to everyday relationships. When it is recognised, though, it becomes difficult for practitioners to manage; their attempts to respect individual patients' autonomy can impinge on their sense of professionalism and their accountability to both the patient and the general public. The Mental Health Act is often involved in coercive practice, which can become a double-edged sword for practitioners: it can be a welcomed mechanism for administering so-called treatment even against patients' wishes, but it can also undermine their relationship with patients.

Dominating medication treatment for voice hearing

Consistent with the views collected from voice hearers in Chapter 3, overwhelmingly, practitioners reported medication as the dominant form of treatment for people who hear voices and an overall medicalisation of voice hearing. Practitioners were critical of the over-reliance on medication within mental health services and the lack of alternative treatment choices available to patients distressed by voice hearing. Some practitioners talked about their frustration with some of their colleagues in their clinical teams, who seldom attempted to support patients in their sense-making of voice hearing. Practitioners reported this leads to a convention wherein practitioners align with a medicalising of voice hearing and patients identify with the diagnoses given to them, typically schizophrenia. Penny, a mental health nurse from the third focus group, reflected on this medicalisation in her comments below, which infers that patients who do not believe their voices are a symptom of an illness such as schizophrenia lack insight:

I think it's very dependent on the patient's level of insight and how motivated they are in terms of acknowledging what's going on and what they can do about it. I have patients on my caseload who have been in service 30, 40 years and they still don't have the insight to be able to work on their shared symptoms and their voices because they don't acknowledge that they're as a result of mental health problems, of schizophrenia, of psychosis; they don't acknowledge that at all.

Despite the above comments, some practitioners held a different view regarding medication. They reflected during discussions that voices serve a purpose in a voice hearers' life, and they recognised that some voice hearers who valued their voices were worried that practitioners would take their voices away through medication. Practitioners also believed that medication could stop patients from thinking clearly or feeling emotions. These practitioners believed that medication had a disempowering effect on voice hearers and their experiences of voice hearing and losing their voices could leave the person feeling lonely and without a sense of purpose or identity. Furthermore, some practitioners said they believed that over-reliance on medication leads patients to perceive they are unable to cope without medication and without their voices. They reported they had observed in patients a cycle of them using medication to take away or quieten their voices, which also led to taking away patients' opportunities to understand their voices. In these situations, practitioners reflected that patients sometimes ask for medication to take away their voices or distress rather than talk about their voices with practitioners or learn how to manage their distress without medication.

Practitioners in the second focus group reflected on a more concerning disempowering and institutionalising effect of over-reliance on medication. They were of the view that medication traps people in mental health services because their risk to self and/or others can be too high for them to be discharged from services. This is captured in the brief conversation below between Jack and Lucy:

Jack: … I'm just on about the predominant thing of what keeps people in mental health services, is medication.

Lucy: And I would probably think that's the first treatment that's offered.

Engaging with voice hearing

Although medication was reported by practitioners to be the dominant method of "treating" voice hearing and related distress (and voice hearers similarly reported this in Chapter 3), practitioners also reflected during focus group discussions on the importance of providing a choice of treatment approaches. Practitioners recognised that some patients do not want to take medication for their voice-related experiences and, instead, valued alternative support such as talking therapies or occupational therapy. However, they were also critical of the lack of resources in mental health services for alternative approaches, especially psychological support, which limits the range of supportive options for people distressed by voice hearing and undermines practitioners' attempts to support them. Instead, practitioners believed the provision of alternative approaches is influenced by individual practitioners' preference rather than broader service-wide provision.

Practitioners from all three focus groups stressed the importance of developing helping relationships with people distressed by voices. Encouragingly, some practitioners were curious and motivated to learn about voice hearing and engage in conversation with people about their experiences of voice hearing. They spoke about the importance of respecting and learning from people about their voice hearing. Jack, from the second focus group, reflected on this:

> As you get more experienced at doing it [Talking with Voices approach] you get more confident over the years. It's alright to ask questions about people's voices. It's alright to ask them about if they've got a name, how old are they, do they come from the inside, do they come from the outside of your head. Or is there anywhere else they come from? And when you do the mapping of where they hear them from as well, you get more used to it, don't you? And you're like oh god, yeah. And it destigmatises it for you as well.

The lack of resources not only related to the range of support available to people distressed by voice hearing but also extended to the clinical supervision and support available to practitioners. This, consequently, impacted the quality of practitioners' clinical practice. For example, some practitioners reported they engaged in the Talking with Voices (TwV) approach. Practitioners in the second focus group reflected on their feelings of anxiety when trying to discuss this approach with a person about their voices and to talk directly with voices. Their lack of training and supervision on this led to this being perceived as an anxiety-provoking and difficult approach to attempt with patients. It also meant that practitioners had limited (if any) opportunities to reflect on their own practice and consider what type of conversations with voices are helpful or unhelpful. We can see this with Rose from focus group three, who recalled her TwV approach with a patient's voice:

> I've coerced with the voices and I've coerced with the patient and I've said to them, would it help if I told your voice to go away… I won't tell you sometimes the terms I say. You've got to talk in a language with your patients that they use… And I've got permission off the patient, and I've spoken to the voice in a coercive manner and I've asked the patient if – a lot of the times it hasn't made a bit of difference, but a few times the patient has said the voice is listening to you and it doesn't want you to be here and it doesn't want you to talk to it.

It is worth reflecting on the above example. Whilst it is encouraging to see this practitioner attempt to engage with voice hearing and support the person by engaging with their voices, it is also important for supportive opportunities to enable deeper consideration about how such approaches might affect the person and their voices. In the above example, there is a risk of replicating coercive approaches through the TwV approach and, thus, inadvertently disempowering the voice hearer (and their voices). With clinical support, practitioners could explore these and similar issues to increase their awareness of these intra- and inter-personal dynamics.

Normalising is a concept widely accepted in mental health literature and practice and is considered a valuable component of a supportive approach. The application of the concept has ranged from normalising voice hearing as a phenomenon experienced by many other people to normalising voice hearing as a natural human experience. These may appear to be similar but reflect different perspectives on voice hearing. The first infers that normalising is the sharing of an experience, regardless of the causation; the latter infers that normalising is literally to experience something normal under particular (and difficult) circumstances. We can see these two different perspectives in two of the focus group discussions. In focus group two, Jack reported that he shares with patients his own experiences of anxiety and rumination. As such, he normalises emotional distress by relating to his own emotions and distress and to something that happens to other people. In focus group three, Naomi offers something similar but extends this by relating voice hearing to an illness:

> Actually this [voice hearing] is normal, this does happen to people quite often, that's why there are teams developed around it, that's what we're here for. And getting them to understand that it's just another illness; it's something that you can recover from, something that you can get better.

Both of these examples reflect practitioners' intent on supporting and empathising with people distressed by voice hearing but Naomi's comment "getting [the patient] to understand it's just another illness", arguably, attributes voice hearing to an illness within a medicalised framework in which voices are considered to be a symptom of, for example, a schizophrenia "illness". The previous code, you may remember, reflected practitioners' belief that medication dominates mental healthcare for voice hearing, which they also believe leads to patients perceiving they are unable to cope with their voices and related distress without medication. Consequently, this approach can disempower voice hearers.

Power is threaded throughout practitioners' reflections on engaging with voice hearing. In addition to the disempowering effect of over-reliance on medication, power can be seen to be represented elsewhere in practitioners' accounts. For example, practitioners in the second focus group reflected on the impact of power on practitioner-patient relationships and how they tried to balance this by respecting patients as equals and individuals and by refraining from imposing their own perspectives onto patients. This can be seen in the following discussion between Ken and Lucy:

Ken: I think you've got to give [patients] enough space to work a lot of things out themselves as well, to come to their own conclusions. I was working with somebody recently and they dropped in there that actually their voices might be related to some anxiety. And I thought that was...they'd come to their own [conclusion]...So we explored that further and the potentials of that and what that meant and the reactions that causes them or the impacts that it might have on them. So yeah, I think it's important not to go in with the full, this is the right explanation, this is... I mean it is a lot of guesswork, isn't it? And it's important that they guess as much as we guess really.

Lucy: And you have experiences, don't you? I did the other day where we were talking to someone about their mental health has deteriorated and I was open and honest about what my thoughts were on that. And then when I asked about [their] voices they were...'no, no. No voices there'. And I felt it was because I was looking at it from a mental health point of view...

The final way practitioners tried to balance power was through their attempts to make sense of voice hearing. Some, such as Penny from group three, would include other people such as family members to help gather as much information as possible about voice hearing. Mary, also from group three, tried to balance power in voice hearing by learning about alternative approaches to the conventional medicalisation of voice hearing and appreciated multiple interpretations. Mary is a nurse who completed further training as a therapist and illustrates the value of supporting practitioners to develop and apply critical thinking when supporting people:

I learnt about never being married to the model. The model is just a model. All these are just ideas, and we offer them out to people, and then they take up what they think is helpful to them. And once I get married to the model and believe that that's the only thing and the right thing then I'm in danger then of cutting off everything else to the person.

Practitioners all stressed the importance of working collaboratively with individual voice hearers, but Mary also stressed the importance of making sense of voice hearing within a family rather than individual context. Some, such as Rose from group three, reflected on the importance of making judgements based on their own observations and interpretations. However, there was less discussion or evidence of practitioners having had opportunities to be reflexive in practice to help disentangle their own interpretations from patients' accounts. For example, a practitioner might believe a person's voice hearing is an illness that requires medication, which might not be a belief shared by that individual. However, we will leave the discussion on a positive note by highlighting the following conversation between Jack and Lucy from the second focus group:

Jack: I think we get away from symptoms, don't we? None of us want to use the word symptoms because I can't stand that. It's not a symptom, it's an experience of someone, isn't it?

Lucy: I don't think we do call them symptoms at all.
Jack: No.
Lucy: We don't as a team. I think it's very much…yeah, factual about what they're… We might make links about it, about what that might mean.

Generally, practitioners do attempt to engage with voice hearing experiences, typically against a backdrop of a dominant biomedical approach in which voice hearing is largely believed to be a symptom of a mental illness and for which medication is conventionally the main if not only approach as a "treatment". Despite this, many practitioners try to find ways alternative to this convention to help understand voice hearing and support people distressed by it. This involves recognition of the role of power in practitioner-patient relationships and ways to attempt to balance this.

Feeling constrained

I cried last week because there's absolutely nothing, absolutely nothing I can do for this lady apart from go and visit once a week. It doesn't matter what I do it's not going to improve her quality of life.

The above quote is from Sarah, an Occupational Therapist from group three. Given the difficulties we have already described regarding coercion, the lack of alternatives to medication, and the challenges of trying to engage with experiences of voice hearing, perhaps, it is unsurprising that practitioners struggle to help. Practitioners overwhelmingly felt constrained in their attempts to understand and support people distressed by voice hearing. They felt the impact resulting from a lack, or in some cases a complete absence, of psychological support in mental health services. This left them feeling unsupported and anxious when trying to support large numbers of patients, especially when trying to understand and support people distressed related to trauma. Some patients with long-standing diagnoses and for which medication had little effect were believed to be "treatment resistant". Practitioners reported they felt particularly helpless in their attempts to support patients, and they became upset at the thought of being unable to help people distressed by voice hearing. This was a difficult tension for practitioners because they acknowledged the importance for them to have opportunities to make positive differences, where they could anticipate "results" with patients they perceived had "recovery potential".

Practitioners across all three focus groups talked at length about feeling constrained in their attempts to support people distressed by voice hearing. Interestingly, much of this is related to their professional accountabilities and being "duty bound" to their professional responsibilities. For example, Lucy from group two was frustrated that practitioners had to "tick boxes…as part of your job". Practitioners reported that valuable meaningful time spent with patients was taken up by completing tasks such as administering depot medications or completing certain clinical assessments required as part of policy within their organisation rather than spending more quality time with people to, for example from Penny in group three, "look at really proactive coping strategies for voices".

So, despite practitioners recognising the importance of "being human" to build their relationships with patients, they felt obliged to perform clinical procedures such as complete standardised assessments, including risk management, within specific timescales and encourage medication compliance to meet their professional responsibilities. Practitioners were cognisant of their perceived pressure to "treat" voice hearers and questioned their colleagues' perceived need to make voices and distress go away. Practitioners also reflected that patients did not always work to the timescales imposed upon them and, sometimes, the provision of treatment or support is for practitioners' "own need for self-gratification". Extending this, practitioners acknowledged the importance of their role of holding onto a belief that they can make a difference for patients. Interestingly, those practitioners from the focus groups who did not have a professional registration, such as Ken from group two, felt "freer" and did not need to "push medication".

Within the context described by practitioners regarding the dominance of medicine, their perceived lack of professional support, and the requirements to "tick boxes", they reflected on feeling nervous about trying alternative approaches, such as TwV. This was further complicated by a perceived hierarchy of power amongst practitioners, wherein medicine dominates as a "treatment" approach and is led by medical practitioners. Those in the second focus group were critical of this and the associated diagnostic-led approach within mental healthcare, which they reported had led to prescribed medication for most patients and, in turn, has led to patients asking for medication rather than considering non-medication approaches. Some practitioners such as Rose in group three managed this by excluding where possible her medical practitioner colleagues in appointments with patients to help provide space to discuss non-medication treatment options. Practitioners also commented on "power differentials" between community and inpatient teams, illustrated by experts from Jack below during his discussion in the second focus group:

> We do go and try and influence [care]... but I guess it feels like at times the power differential between us and the wards... that's when it becomes conflictual and... the [patient] always seems to get forgotten I think.

Practitioners reflected that this power difference results in differences or gaps in treatment approaches between different teams but within the same healthcare organisation, which ultimately results in disjointed treatment experiences for patients. Community-based practitioners in the focus group reflected that community-based approaches to voice hearing typically paused when a patient was admitted to an inpatient unit, leading to inpatient practitioners' "insulating" parts of a voice hearers experiences rather than exploring the related distress. It matters greatly to practitioners to support patients and hold a belief that they can make positive differences for people in distress, both generally in terms of their emotional well-being and, specifically, in terms of voice hearing. They try to do this but feel constrained against a backdrop of numerous challenges, leading to a feeling of disempowerment in terms of helping people distressed by voice hearing.

Privileging practitioners' interpretations

In Chapter 3, we reported that during the interviews, voice hearers reflected on their lack of agency in terms of their struggle to influence their voices and their treatment decisions and the negative impact of this on their voice and treatment-related experiences. Furthermore, they reflected on the dominant narratives within mental health services that "treat" voice hearing with medication and, consequently, align voice hearing with a largely biomedical perspective. Their reported experiences are consistent with those reported by practitioners during the focus group discussions. It was evident from the focus groups that practitioners can have a dominant influence over voice hearing experiences through their sharing with voice hearers of their "professional" perspective when making sense of voices and their subsequent administration of medication as the mainstay method of addressing problems related to voice hearing.

Practitioners reflected on their power over patients. They spoke about their awareness of the consequences for patients should they refuse interventions. For example, should a patient living at home or in the community refuse treatment, they could be recalled under the Mental Health Act back into hospital to receive treatment. Contributing to practitioners' power is their collective team approach. Practitioners held regular team meetings in which they shared information about patients and in which they would make and agree on collective decisions about interventions, such as a plan to administer an enforced injection of medication. From a professional perspective, it was important to reach a team decision but it also, inadvertently, strengthened interpretations and subsequent "treatment" approaches according to practitioners' perspectives and at the exclusion of voice hearers' interpretations or considerations.

Practitioners also reflected during focus group discussions that, typically, their peers understood voice hearing based on their observations of patients, their assumptions about voice hearing and they subsequently would decide what they thought was best for patients distressed by voices. Their decisions lacked sufficient acknowledgement of patients' expertise regarding their own voice hearing experiences. Debbie from the first focus group reflected on this:

> [Patients] scream bloody murder that they don't want this medication. But yet as a clinical team there's been a decision made that in the best interests of that person at that time [to give medication], because they are incapacitated, and they're so unwell.

This contributed to a notion that practitioners "know best" even though, as practitioners reflected, their understanding and subsequent interventions regarding voice hearing were based on a professional perspective as we commented above. Beth, from the first focus group, reflected that this perspective considers voice hearing from a "mental health point of view", which is informed by practitioners engaging in professional education and literature. Despite some attempts by practitioners to use patients' language rather than professional language, practitioners reported that there was generally a lack of appreciation by their peers of structural power broadly within mental healthcare and its influence on informing professional education and shaping practitioner observations and understanding of voice hearing. For example, for some practitioners, it was important to determine whether the person's voice hearing was "true and valid", whether voices were heard from inside or outside of a person's head, or whether the person had their own thoughts. For practitioners, information such as this informed their perception of whether voices were linked to trauma or whether the person dissociated or even "truly" heard voices. Some practitioners, such as Jack from the second focus group, were critical of this "mental health perspective" and of mental health services for being too diagnostic-led. Jack reflected:

> I don't think it's a diagnostic thing like schizophrenia. I don't believe in that label... it's a way of coping with life. And I think there's a lot of metaphor in voice hearing, for what people experience... even though the voices might be negative, they're actually maybe helping keeping them safe.

Jack was concerned that people who hear voices are typically diagnosed with schizophrenia, then prescribed a psychotropic medication, which leads to that person perceiving they are unable to cope with their voices or related stress without the medication. In other words, it can be disempowering for voice hearers.

These discussions from the practitioners' focus groups reflect an imbalance of power between people aiming to provide support and people experiencing distress related to voice hearing. Despite examples in which they acknowledged a patient's perspective and experience relating to voice hearing, mostly professional agendas shaped the conventional understanding and "treatment" approach within mental health services.

Struggling to know how to support voice hearing

It may be a surprise to some readers to learn that many practitioners find it difficult to know how to engage in a meaningful way with patients about their voice hearing. Practitioners spoke about these difficulties during the focus groups and several reasons were revealed. They spoke about historical and cultural beliefs within mental health teams that have largely led to the dismissal of the importance of understanding an individual's personal meaning associated with their voice hearing. As such, practitioners reflected that sometimes their peers discouraged them from talking to people about their voices for fear of colluding with voice hearing. Practitioners from the second focus group were especially critical of their peers within mental health services for continually failing to genuinely listen to people about their voices and avoiding discussions about voice hearing with patients for fear of collusion. However, it is important to highlight examples from Debbie and Fiona, both from the first focus group, who reflected on the value of listening to people about their voice hearing and trying to offer reassurance. Debbie reflected:

> I think there's sometimes a bit of comfort in somebody that is actually listening and validating them, if you're listening to what they're saying about their voices, rather than dismissing it.
>
> (Debbie, group 1)

And Fiona reflected:

> Sometimes we get people hearing that they're an awful person, getting told all these horrible things. And I think sometimes it's just...I know people have said that it's nice just to get that reassurance that they're not...when they tell you what they're experiencing you can try and help them work through it a bit. Maybe saying well, you know, you're not an awful person.

During focus group discussions, some practitioners reported that many of their peers struggled to know how to have a conversation about voice hearing and felt anxious about speaking to patients about their voices for fear of making things worse. This led to them avoiding these discussions. Sometimes, practitioners became concerned about patients to the extent that they would exclude them from ward-based interventions such as occupational therapy. Jack and Lucy, from the second group, reflected on this:

Jack: People can't deal with distress. They can't deal with somebody else's distress...We haven't got a tolerance for someone's distress.

Lucy: And then what does that say? It's about all emotional regulation stuff, that we can't deal with that. We're trying to stop your emotions, when actually we need to be teaching people more about how to manage their own distress and know that it's alright to be really sad and really happy or whatever.

Practitioners revealed that, generally, either they themselves and/or their peers lacked confidence, knowledge, and expertise regarding how they can help people distressed by voice hearing. Instead, practitioners would focus on managing side effects, such as anxiety, associated with voice hearing or avoid further exploration of voice hearing and encourage distraction from the voices, illustrated by Sarah from the third focus group:

> So, rather than asking him and distressing him by what they were saying, because he would never tell me, and he'd say you know because they're actually talking to you because I can hear them, so he could hear the voices talking

to me, but I would just say are they inside your head or outside. And then that would give me an aim to say, okay let's distract that. Whereas if they were inside his head I'd just leave them because he was quite happy with those voices.

Given these challenges experienced by practitioners, it may not surprise you to learn that practitioners also found it difficult to encourage patients to disclose information about their voice hearing. This issue came up in all three focus group discussions, where practitioners had either experienced themselves or observed their peers struggle to collect voice-related information from patients. The practitioners attributed patients' reluctance to disclose information to their fear of potential consequences; for example, practitioners suggested a patient might worry that their disclosure of voice hearing might lead to practitioner concerns and eventual hospitalisation (or restrictions of some sort). Interestingly, practitioners did not demonstrate any self-awareness during their reflections concerning whether their own fears might actually discourage patients from talking about their voice hearing experiences.

Summary

So, what sense can we make of these findings? Well, it is quite clear from practitioners' reports that they too believe medication is perceived as a "treatment" for voice hearing and related distress and, overwhelmingly, is the most available (and administered) form of treatment. They also acknowledged that a lack of resources effectively means that many patients are excluded from alternative approaches such as talking therapies or TwV. Practitioners also reflected that medication is largely inseparable from coercion. They generally first try softer coercive approaches, such as persuasion, to encourage patients to accept the medication but, where this fails, they administer increasingly harder coercive approaches to enforce medication, for example through the application of the Mental Health Act and/or physically enforcing medication compliance. It is also clear from practitioners' discussions that they experience coercion as paradoxically both helpful and harmful. They valued the use of coercion when they 'needed' to administer medication, for example, but they also recognised it to be a hindrance when forming relationships with patients. As such, they felt conflicted and constrained. To complicate this further, practitioners also found it difficult to determine whether their practice was coercive and, where they do recognise it as coercion, it was important for them to justify it and, preferably, to soften the coercion and reduce the impact on patients.

Another key point to recap from these findings is that, in addition to coercion, practitioners contribute to their power over patients by privileging their own perspectives and agenda over patients, leading to a situation in which the "practitioner knows best". This typically influences treatment decisions. However, interestingly, there was lack of evidence from practitioners' discussions to suggest they are cognizant of their own lack of agency in terms of shaping treatment approaches.

Finally, a key point on which to leave this chapter and pave the way for us to address in Chapter 5 is the struggle practitioners typically experience in their efforts to help voice hearers. Many do not feel confident nor have sufficient knowledge to engage meaningfully with people's experiences of voice hearing. As such, largely, they do two things. They avoid meaningful discussions about voice hearing and, instead, focus on the side effects of symptoms of voice hearing such as anxiety. They also normalise voice hearing experiences but seldom attempt to disentangle their own beliefs from this nor contextualise the impact of a broader biomedical narrative on how voice hearers and practitioners come to understand voice hearing and the subsequent treatment approaches. In Chapter 5, we will bring together the findings from the individual interviews in Chapter 3 and the focus group discussions reported in this chapter.

Chapter 5

We're in it together

Understanding voice hearing through a tripartite voice hearer-voice practitioner relationship

We have explored the reported experiences of people who hear voices and from practitioners who support people distressed by voices. We now bring these reported experiences together. If you would like to read more about how the analyses of these reported experiences were synthesised, please go to the appendix at the back of the book where you can find a more detailed description. Synthesising these experiences led to the completion of the Tripartite Relationship Theory of voice hearing, comprising the following themes:

1 Personal bully;
2 Interpersonal dynamic (extent of collaboration; acknowledging or avoiding voices);
3 Who's making sense (dominant narratives; collective search for meaning);
4 Medication: helping or hindering (agreement on its purpose; control over treatment decisions; lack of alternative);
5 Level of agency (constrained by coercion; varying ability to influence change).

Although we recognise that voice hearing is a personal experience specific for the person hearing the voices, this theory proposes that voice hearing experiences within a mental healthcare context involve voice hearers, their voices, and practitioners. Whereas previous research and literature has focused on relationships between voice hearers (or patients) and practitioners and relationships between voice hearers and their voices, to our knowledge this is the first study to have focused on a tripartite relationship between voice hearers, voices, and practitioners. In other words, there are both intra-personal relationships (between the voice hearer and their voices) and inter-personal relationships (between the voice hearer and practitioners) that influence voice hearing experiences. Figure 5.1 illustrates the five interdependent themes of the theory to represent challenges both voice hearers and practitioners similarly experience regarding their perceived lack of power, their struggle to relate with voices, their struggle to make sense of voice hearing, and the extent to which medication helps or hinders voice hearing. Additionally, both influencing and influenced by this are the way in which people experience their voices, which is typically of a bullying nature.

DOI: 10.4324/9781032619910-7

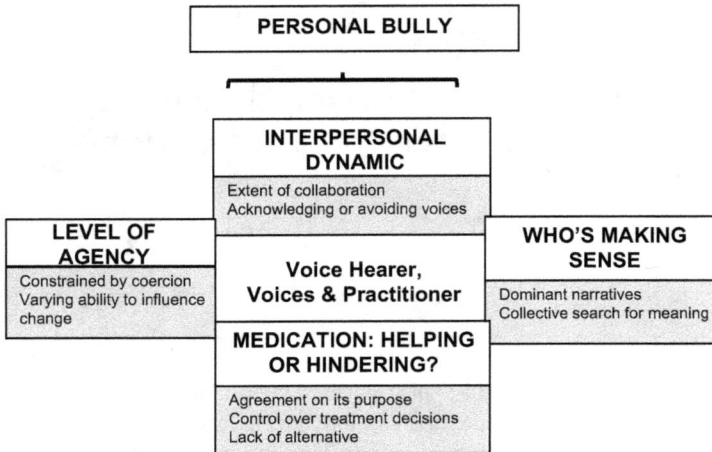

Figure 5.1 Tripartite relationship theory of voice hearing.

Now that we have explained how the final development of the theory was completed, we will now explain each of the themes in detail.

Personal bully

This is uniquely experienced solely by voice hearers. The personal bully typically appears before a person distressed by voice hearing first presents to mental health services but usually continues beyond this and impacts on the tripartite relationship through both influencing, and being influenced by, the other four themes. You may remember from Chapter 3 that we identified from the interviews with people talking about their voice hearing that there were two key elements to this. First, the personal bully represented experiences of being persecuted by voices. People may experience a range of different voices, and indeed some voices might be considered to provide a positive experience and be welcomed by the voice hearer. However, the personal bully represents the voices that are distressing and of a persecutory nature. Second, this theme also encapsulates voices that don't like the voice hearer getting help and, consequently, whenever the voice hearer tries to engage in something that might be beneficial in some way for themselves, the voices respond in ways that the voice hearer finds distressing. Please go back to Chapter 3 if you would like to remind yourself of the details.

Finally, the personal bully can be positively changed through the voice hearer's increased level of agency, their development of more effective and supportive relationships, through finding a meaningful explanation of voice hearing, and through the voice hearer taking more control regarding if and how they use medication. These can change how voice hearers experience their voices to the extent that they can perceive them to become more supportive, even protective.

Interpersonal dynamic

The remaining four themes concern not just voice hearers and their voices but also practitioners. Collectively, these four themes impact the "personal bully". The interpersonal dynamic theme encapsulates complex interpersonal interactions between voice hearers and practitioners whilst, simultaneously, the voice hearer either interacts with their voices, concentrates on avoiding interacting, or observes or hears interactions between different voices. Unsurprisingly, these interactions can contribute towards a complex, chaotic, and stressful relational context both internally and externally for voice hearers. They can also contribute towards a challenge for practitioners, who might typically try to determine how to engage with and support the voice hearer.

i Extent of collaboration

Both voice hearers and practitioners can find it difficult to talk about voices, which can lead them to either minimise or even completely avoid meaningful engagement regarding voice hearing. Despite this being an important element for many people to address voice-related distress, this lack (or complete avoidance) of talking can leave voice hearers and practitioners with contrasting, and possibly even conflicting, perceptions of each other's intentions. For example, influenced by their voices, voice hearers might be fearful that practitioners want them to confess their voice hearing and disclose information about their voices, which can lead to further reactions from their voices (such as anger, aggression or anxiety) and increasingly distressing voice content or activity. By contrast, however, practitioners might believe voice hearers conceal their voices due to a mental illness, become concerned about the risks they associate with voices and, consequently, want to reduce this through medicating the voice hearer.

Of key importance here is the degree to which both voice hearers and practitioners work together towards the same goal. The more voice hearers and practitioners can understand and reach an agreement on the purpose of support and treatment and collaborate with one another, the more likely this will contribute towards reducing voice-related distress.

ii Acknowledging or avoiding voices

The quality of the interpersonal dynamic can vary, depending on the extent to which voices are acknowledged or avoided. In terms of avoidance, voice hearers might assume that practitioners avoid talking to them about their voices; however, practitioners might struggle to know how to meaningfully talk about (and with) voices. By contrast, practitioners might assume voice hearers are reluctant to talk about their voices, or even disclose their voice hearing. We know from previous research that talking about voices can be difficult for both voice hearers (Bogen Johnston et al., 2020) and practitioners (Harris & Panozzo, 2019; McMullan et al., 2018; Coffey & Hewitt, 2008). We also know from this study that practitioners can struggle to know how to positively impact on distressing voice hearing experiences. Typically, they instead focus on managing emotional reactions (or symptoms) to voice hearing, such as anxiety, through their administration of medication. So, whereas voice hearers might emotionally distance or distract themselves from their voices, practitioners also distance themselves through their avoidance of direct engagement in voice hearing and their reliance on medication for symptom management.

In terms of poor quality regarding the interpersonal dynamic, and thus negatively impacting voice hearing experiences, voice hearers can experience and struggle in mutually hostile and critical relationships with their voices. Typically, they may desperately want to get rid of their voices and, as mentioned above, believe that practitioners either fail to engage with them about their voice hearing or fail to provide sufficient support for their voice hearing. However, practitioners can also struggle. They can lack confidence in terms of meaningfully engaging in and understanding voice hearing experiences and so, typically, can focus on voice hearers' emotional (i.e., anxiety) and behavioural (i.e., social withdrawal) reactions to distressing voices.

Better quality regarding the interpersonal dynamic involves more positive engagement between voice hearers and practitioners. For voice hearers, this involves relating more positively with their voices to reduce distress associated with their voices and feeling more valued and supported by practitioners. For practitioners, this involves becoming more curious to talk to voice hearers about voice hearing through a greater emphasis on building supportive relationships to enable the development of more meaningful and helpful conversations.

Finally, voice hearers' and practitioners' levels of perceived agency (more about this shortly) also influence the interpersonal dynamic. Voice hearers who feel less threatened and controlled by their voices and who feel more involved in treatment decisions about their own health will typically find it less difficult to be with their voices and with practitioners and feel less fearful of disclosing their voices to practitioners. However, this is also influenced by practitioners' interpersonal qualities in terms of being genuinely collaborative, their ability to genuinely listen to people about their experiences, and to engage meaningfully with voice hearing experiences.

Who's making sense?

Understanding why a person hears voices and how they experience voice hearing is important in terms of if and how they accept voices, how they subsequently live with them and the support they might need. Both voice hearers and practitioners might make sense of voice hearing, or at least attempt to, from a range of sources and sometimes even the same source, such as literature. However, as we discussed in the previous theme, there can sometimes be a lack of collaboration between the two when attempting to make sense. A consequence of this lack of working in partnership is a prevailing influence of professional (practitioner) explanations of voice hearing. Dillon and Hornstein (2013) argue that a dominant psychiatric narrative constructs people as "chronic" or "treatment-resistant", despite it being the medication (rather than the person) failing to prevent distressing voices. So, of key importance here is *how* voice hearing is understood and *who* influences this understanding. Furthermore, there is a potentially empowering act of constructing meaning and making sense of one's own experiences and, ideally in terms of a clinical context, through supportive relationships with practitioners.

i Dominant narratives

Making sense of voice hearing is inextricably linked with power, both within individuals and relationships within clinical contexts as illustrated through the tripartite relationship theory, but also within broader social, political, and cultural contexts. This shapes the narrative about voice hearing. For example, developing an understanding of voice hearing can be influenced by voice hearers' beliefs and their subsequent interpretations of their experiences, by the voices themselves in terms of their content and their presence, and by practitioners' beliefs and their subsequent influence on people who hear voices. And, of course, this can be extended more broadly across a range of different contexts in our societies in terms of the range of beliefs about voice hearing. Typically, many people distressed by voices believe, through listening to what their voices say and how they speak/communicate, that their voices are omniscient and omnipotent and are an all-powerful presence for which they have no control.

However, voice hearers' and practitioners' understanding of voice hearing is typically developed against a backdrop of mental healthcare in which a dominant biomedical model shapes an illness narrative about voice hearing. This leads to a prevailing belief within mental healthcare that voice hearing is a symptom of a mental illness and requires treatment in the form of medication. Consequently, the importance of and connection between voice hearing and life experiences is marginalised. Instead, through more effective collaboration, voice hearers and practitioners can explore different narratives that influence the understanding of voice hearing and the influence of these on how voices are understood.

ii Collective search for meaning

We previously reported to have found that both people distressed by voices and practitioners trying to provide support can struggle to know how to reduce voice-related distress. How both make sense of voices may not always be in synchrony with one another and, consequently, practitioners can form an understanding of voices without sufficient meaningful engagement with voice hearers. As we commented above, this can contribute towards a professional (and conventional) narrative about voice hearing that can marginalise other, less conventional narratives.

Consequently, it is important for practitioners and voice hearers to establish some collective endeavour in making sense of voices. Both can struggle to disentangle their own contributions when trying to make sense of voice hearing; voice hearers, for example, might struggle to disentangle their emotions (largely fear and anxiety), whereas practitioners might struggle to disentangle their professional interpretations. Failure to collaborate effectively with one another can lead to a privileging of dominant narratives, which typically fail to sufficiently consider an individual's voice hearing experience, and also a situation in which practitioners typically develop a shared understanding of voices not with the individual voice hearer but with their professional colleagues. As such, important to the process of reducing voice-related distress is to identify power relations in determining *who* makes sense of voice hearing and *how* this is informed.

Medication: helping or hindering?

As we reported in the previous two chapters, both voice hearers and practitioners experienced medication overwhelmingly as the primary intervention for voice-related distress. In fact, rather than considering whether to use medication, the real option tended to be concerned with deciding on the specific medication and how much dosage. Two key issues regarding medication are, first, to determine whether it actually helps a person with their experience of voice hearing or whether it hinders their experience and, second, for practitioners and voice hearers to agree on how best to use it. This latter point must be considered in a context of varying and, typically, limited treatment options and include the possibility that an individual may wish to stop medication altogether.

  i Agreement on its purpose

    Voice hearers and practitioners have complex relationships with medication and mixed experiences of using it. Both generally perceive some benefit from using medication but also believe it can be harmful and difficult to stop using it. Although voice hearers might receive some relief from voice-related distress from using medication, they typically find it has insufficient impact on the presence and content of voices and it causes unwanted side effects. Similarly, practitioners are reliant upon medication as an intervention and assume it reduces a person's voice-related distress, but they also acknowledge longer term consequences of using it (i.e., dependency, side effects, and stigma associated with taking medication). As such, it is important for both to understand how medication impacts voice hearing experiences and to reach agreement on how best to use it, if at all. A key challenge in doing this is to develop confidence and sufficient agency to address distressing voice hearing through an approach that is effective and meaningful for the voice hearer, which includes agreement on the purpose of using medication (and whether to use medication at all).

  ii Control over treatment decisions

    In terms of whether to use medication, a key issue is the extent of control one has over the decision to use it (or not use it). There is a body of literature in which the importance of patient involvement is recognised, but in which it is also acknowledged that power relations and coercion influence decisions, and that patients' and practitioners' perceptions can differ regarding the extent to which treatment decisions are shared. As we have reported from the interviews and focus group discussions in Chapters 3 and 4, respectively, voice hearers felt disempowered regarding decisions about their own treatment, including medication, and practitioners felt disempowered in terms of influencing some treatment decisions, particularly medication. Extending this point, voice hearers may wish to reduce their medication or even stop using it altogether but, generally, receive insufficient support from practitioners to do so. However, similarly, practitioners generally feel unsupported by their colleagues to help voice hearers reduce or stop using medication.

Furthermore, medication is entangled with power or, more specifically in terms of the tripartite relationship theory, a perceived lack of agency (discussed below). It can exert a power over both voice hearers and practitioners in terms of dependency on using it, either taking it or administering it (and, consequently, trapping voice hearers in mental health services longer term). For example, voices can comment on medication and either encourage or discourage the voice hearer to take it; voice hearers know that practitioners can enforce medication; and practitioners know that changing or stopping medication for a voice hearer is, typically, beyond their influence. Indeed, both voice hearers and practitioners recognise that medication is often accepted because of a combination of practitioners' persuasion and voice hearers' fear that refusal can lead to an escalation from verbal persuasion to physical enforcement.

iii Lack of alternative

The extent to which a range of supportive interventions is available greatly influences experiences of voice hearing. Unfortunately, though, there is a general lack of choice in mental healthcare for people distressed by voice hearing. As commented above, voice hearers and practitioners perceive their options relate to the type and dosage of medication rather than genuine choice of alternatives. As we have discussed throughout this and the previous two chapters, in a treatment context in which medication is heavily relied upon and in which there can often be insufficient meaningful collaboration between practitioners and voice hearers, both can become reliant on medication and lack confidence in the availability of options for alternative support or interventions.

Level of agency

Situated within a broader context of psychiatry, this theme impacts voice hearing experiences through the involvement of dynamic relations involving power, control, and influence between voice hearers, their voices, and practitioners. According to Hearn, power concentrates in particular areas and within a "web of relations" (p.9) and hierarchies, which can usefully be applied to the Tripartite Relationship Theory. This reflects an asymmetrical rather than balanced distribution of power within the voice hearer-voice practitioner relationship. As derived from the interview and focus group discussions, in terms of power, the level of agency can be greater in one area of the tripartite relationship than another. For example, an individual may perceive they have some degree of influence over their prescribed medication, i.e., they may choose whether they take it, or they may be able to reach agreement with their clinical team regarding their prescription, but they may perceive they have no control over their voices. By contrast, a practitioner may perceive they can influence the medication, i.e., they might be a prescriber or have influence on prescribing within their team but have no influence on the impact of voices on the individual.

i Constrained by coercion
In Chapter 2, we asserted that mental healthcare is inextricably intertwined with coercion through a range of softer to harder coercive approaches administered by practitioners. Previous research evidence has focused predominantly on an individual-centric approach to understand coercion, for example through investigating patients' or practitioners' experiences of coercion. Less attention has previously been given in the wider literature to the effect of coercion on interpersonal relationships between voice hearers and practitioners and none specifically concerning coercion between voice hearers and their voices. The interviews with voice hearers revealed that their overall experience of coercion involves their perceptions that both their voices and practitioners can be coercive.

We have seen from the findings of the interviews and focus group discussions that not only does coercion pervade mental healthcare, but also it can be challenging for both voice hearers and practitioners. Voice hearers can experience their voices and practitioners as coercive and controlling and so, typically, perceive they are disempowered in their relationships with voices and practitioners and lack control regarding their treatment. They believe their voices and practitioners can make credible threats towards them and which the voices and practitioners will enact upon unless the voice hearer responds to the threat. By definition this is coercive. However, feeling coerced is not restricted only to voice hearers. Whereas voice hearers might feel marginalised, disempowered, and coerced by voices and practitioners, practitioners can experience similar feelings within their own mental healthcare hierarchy, in which they believe they are expected to administer coercive approaches when needed. Importantly, again as we discussed in Chapter 2 regarding coercion, it is the perception of coercion and how it is administered that influences relationships more than coercion per se.

Regarding the perception of coercion, the findings from the focus group discussions revealed that practitioners can find it difficult to differentiate between coercion and choice. Where they might believe they offer choice, voice hearers might experience this as coercion. For example, a practitioner might believe they provide choice when explaining potential consequences should a patient refuse their prescribed oral medication. So, if a voice hearer refuses to accept oral medication from a practitioner, typically the practitioner responds by explaining their refusal will likely lead to sanctions such as (perhaps further) restrictions to periods of time off the ward (if they are on a ward), a recall back into hospital (if they are living at home or in the community), or even an enforced injection of the medication. Whereas a practitioner might believe this is providing choice, a voice hearer will typically believe this is an actionable threat and, therefore, coercive.

In terms of the level of agency, power relations within the tripartite relationship are not static between voice hearers, their voices, and practitioners but are fluid and, therefore, changeable. For example, voice hearers typically mitigate their distressing voices by complying or by compromising their behaviour in some way in response to voices; practitioners can also comply or compromise through their mitigation of coercion by either justifying their actions or they might incrementally decrease or increase their administration of coercion (e.g., first they might apply softer versions of coercion such as persuasion, then negotiation, then more explicit threats to avoid harder versions of coercion such as physical force). However, both have the potential to change their responses in these situations and, therefore, change their levels of agency and the consequential impact on voice hearing experiences.

ii Varying ability to influence change
The extent to which voice hearers and practitioners can influence change, i.e., their level of agency contributes towards the level of voice-related stress and, thus, can change the voice hearing experience. Whereas voice hearers benefit from practitioners with higher levels of agency (i.e., think independently of a prevailing biomedical approach to voice hearing and can bring about change through their actions), practitioners similarly find it less challenging when supporting voice hearers who also have higher levels of agency (i.e., resist commands made by their voices). Practitioners who believe they can bring about positive change can positively influence the way voice hearers might begin to address their own power imbalances, such as increasing their perceived level of agency with their voices, with other practitioners, and in terms of their treatment and related decisions.

However, voice hearers generally believe they lack sufficient ability to influence their voices and their treatment and practitioners generally believe they are constrained in their desire to provide effective support (for example, a lack of alternative options as discussed above) and lack sufficient expertise to reduce voice-related distress. So, whereas voice hearers might wish for something to help make their voices become less distressing or even stop completely, practitioners wish for more professional resources or support to help improve their understanding or level of expertise to reduce voice-related distress. As such, voice hearers can feel helpless in their attempts to cope with their voices, but practitioners can also feel helpless in their efforts to help voice hearers cope with their voices.

Let us again return to Hearn (2012), who conceptualised a reference grid comprising five sets of pairs of terms that encapsulate social power. In his first set of terms, Hearn contrasts physical and social power. Both the voice hearers and practitioners recognised physical power through either receiving or administering physical restraint and enforced medication. More interesting, however, is how the concept of social power relates to voice hearers' experiences. Hearn describes social power as the "application of some invisible force" (p. 5), which usefully explains how voice hearers might perceive voices as having the ability to carry out their threats. For practitioners, it might also explain how they perceive their senior peers to have the ability to influence their application of their professional responsibilities. As you will have likely identified from the information extracted from the interviews, voice hearers mostly described examples of either their voices or practitioners exercising power over them. This was typically in the form of physical enforcement (in the case of practitioners) or issuing verbal threats to bring about an action of some sort (in the case of both practitioners and voices). Power is also described as a relational concept in the sense that an individual's ability to exercise power is structured by social relations (Pansardi, 2012). You may also remember from chapter three that voice hearers described power relations between different voices. For example, one voice might assert dominance over other voices, which can cause distress for the voice hearer.

Summarising the Tripartite Relationship Theory of Voice Hearing

Through the Tripartite Relationship Theory, it is proposed that voice hearing experiences within mental healthcare are best understood through a relational context involving the voice hearer, their voices, and practitioners. This challenges conventional mental healthcare in which the spotlight is predominantly, if not exclusively, focused on individual intrapersonal contexts. Indeed, much of the literature concerning voice hearing has taken an individual-centric approach to understanding predominantly voice hearers' internal context but with less attention given to their external relational context. As such, it challenges practitioners to move away from conceptualising voice hearing solely "within" the individual voice hearer. The conventional approach in mental healthcare also relies on practitioners' expertise to "treat" people distressed by voice hearing and for voice hearers to accept their support. However, practitioners can struggle to reach a sufficient level of expertise to effectively support people distressed by voice hearing and it implies an expectation for voice hearers to accept practitioners' level of expertise and approaches. This approach also largely excludes practitioners from voice hearing experiences.

By moving away from such an approach in which understanding voice hearing has involved too much emphasis placed on voice hearers' inner world experiences, greater recognition is given to their interpersonal relations involving practitioners. Consequently, this broadens the spotlight to include practitioners in voice hearing contexts and supports the notion that improving experiences of voice hearing involves addressing challenges within relationships involving voice hearers, voices, and practitioners.

The five themes that collectively form the theory contribute towards an active and changeable tripartite relationship that influences voice hearing experiences. Encapsulated within this are fluid movements of power and control between voice hearers, voices, and practitioners. This can become a positive energy within the tripartite relationship whereby voice hearing experiences can improve by increasing voice hearers' and practitioners' levels of agency, collaboratively exploring ways to engage with voice hearing, developing meaningful understandings of voices, and identifying and reaching agreement on decisions regarding the role for medication (including deciding if it is needed at all). Such an approach acknowledges that power struggles, interpersonal challenges, developing knowledge and establishing agreed decisions are important to the experience of voice hearing and present challenges within a relational context that involves voice hearers, voices, and practitioners.

Including practitioners in the conceptualisation of voice hearing experiences extends their role and responsibility of providing support by firmly placing them as part of the process of recovery. As such, just as voice hearers must do, practitioners must attend to their own levels of agency and reflect on their own knowledge, beliefs, and expertise. If practitioners wish to be of genuine therapeutic value to voice hearers in reducing their voice-related distress, they must reflect on how they can positively influence change, how they can be interpersonally effective, how they can support people to make their own sense of their own voices, and collaboratively determine whether medication helps or hinders voice hearing experiences. Voice hearers are expected to undertake change to help their own recovery. We have similar expectations of practitioners. They, too, must change if they are to be of therapeutic value in the process of voice hearers' recovery. In Part 3, we will extend this discussion to offer suggestions for making changes to reduce voice-related distress.

Part 3

Putting the Tripartite Relationship Theory into practice

In Part 2, we described how the Tripartite Relationship Theory was developed and we explained how it provides a theoretical explanation for voice hearing experiences within a mental healthcare context. We concluded the previous chapter with a challenge to people distressed by voice hearing and, importantly, also to practitioners working to provide support. We also extend this to any supporter of a person distressed by voice hearing. We urge voice hearers, practitioners, and all supporters to reflect on their own interpersonal effectiveness, their beliefs regarding voice hearing and supportive approaches, broadly, but medication specifically, and their levels of agency in terms of their influence on voice hearing.

In this final part of the book, we discuss how voice hearers, practitioners, and supporters of voice hearers can undertake change to address each of these areas. We recognise that people (voice hearers, practitioners, family, and friends) want to make a positive difference in voice-related distress, but many can find it difficult to do so. Many can find it difficult to talk about voice hearing, for a variety of reasons as we have discussed in previous chapters. It is important to state that the recommendations we make throughout this book are not intended to replace formal therapy. Instead, we hope they provide guidance for people distressed by voice hearing and their supporters (be it practitioners, family, or friends) and enhance any current supportive approaches. It is also important to restate that voice hearing, and subsequent approaches to support difficulties related to it, is complex. It would, therefore, be folly to pretend we can isolate difficulties so easily that we might wish to change. Instead, multiple changes may be required and on multiple levels, ranging from changes at an individual level to changes on a service or policy level (and beyond). Although we focus on recommendations at an individual level in this book, we also argue for the need for change at broader policy and service levels.

At the policy level, we believe there is a continuing need for policy to shape wider societal views about voice hearing. Rather than a portrayal driven by a conventional biological narrative of voice hearing as a symptom of a disease or illness, we believe voice hearing is a normal and understandable response to difficult life experiences; we argue throughout this book that voice hearing for many people has meaning rooted in the life history of the hearer. Contributing towards this, we also believe there is a need to develop educational strategies aimed at

DOI: 10.4324/9781032619910-8

supporting pre- and post-registration practitioners to understand voice hearing. This should include an understanding of how power, and power imbalances, permeate relationships at intra- and inter-personal levels and impact supportive/ treatment approaches. Extending this point, curricula content across professional programmes should support pre- and post-registration practitioners to develop the ability to identify and change barriers within clinical environments to enable more balanced power within these relationships.

At the service level, power imbalances within healthcare organisations need to be tackled. We urge healthcare organisations to take action to address the culture within their organisation, including professional hierarchies, with the aim of reducing coercion. They could develop strategies to facilitate practitioners to routinely engage in critically reflexive discussion and practice regarding relational power. This would also be with the aim of positively influencing shared decision-making concerning supportive approaches and treatment, especially concerning situations in which practitioners and voice hearers might disagree.

Voice hearers may choose or become subject to interventions from mental health services. In a crisis, a voice hearer can feel so disempowered that they can either self-isolate or submit to the commands of voices. The Tripartite Relationship Theory can be useful to help identify aspects of supportive approaches and interventions that can have a positive impact. The way a voice hearer is treated can have a huge impact on how voices respond to the use or misuse of power and can exacerbate or quell distress in the moment. Voices will respond to power imbalance and even subtle coercion by magnifying their own energic capacity to coerce through louder and more distressing use of language and thus increasing the distress to the voice hearer. This creates a tremendous disharmony internally for voice hearers and this is reflected in the disharmony that can develop between the voice hearer and practitioners. Compassionate and informed approaches to voice hearers, where their rights to choice and respect, are the most potent interventions because they offer an antidote to their internal struggle and disempowerment. The careful respect of the voice hearer and the offer of as much mutual power sharing as possible in the choices of services and support for their current distress can help to hold a voice hearer's dignity and the permission for self-agency even if they don't experience the right or capacity to exercise self-agency themselves.

Examples of ways practitioners and supporters can make a positive contribution to the nature of a voice hearer's experience are explored in Part 3 of this book. Above all, practitioners need to be conscious of the fact that they represent a powerful organisation that can cause fear and suspicion for voices hearers and their voices. The quality of empathic and curious conversation can significantly lower voices sense of threat and whilst it rarely eliminates turbulence immediately, it can start a positive and reciprocal relationship that allows voices to emerge and a compassionate space for a voice hearer to start making sense of their voice hearing and establish more harmonious relationships with them.

Putting the recommendations into action

The Tripartite Relationship Theory sets out the broad framework in which we encourage people to make sense of voice hearing and inform approaches to improve voice hearing experiences. We discuss how we utilise this in the delivery of our voice hearing workshops in the remaining chapters of the book.

In Chapter 6, we discuss voice profiling as a way of collating characteristics of voices, which can help begin to establish a sense of order to voice hearing experiences. However, by no means a linear process, this leads us to Chapter 7 where we discuss mapping. This involves plotting a life history of the voice hearer to explore any possible roots to voice hearing experiences. It also involves the application of the Voice Dialogue technique (Stone & Stone, 1989) to map different energies and then an explanation regarding how we utilise this to map different voices. In Chapter 8, we discuss how we can enhance communication between people and their voices. This involves talking directly with voices and mark-making as two approaches we utilise in our work to help communicate with voices to explore ways of understanding voice hearing experiences and reducing voice-related distress. We then turn our attention to Chapter 9 to helping relationships and voice hearing, where we make recommendations informed by the Tripartite Relationship Theory. Finally, we conclude this book with our recommendations for moving forward with voice hearing experiences.

Chapter 6

Phases of voice hearing and voice profiling

We have suggested several important points regarding voice hearing and relationships. These concern the importance of engaging with voices to improve relationships with them, of being aware that relationships develop at both intra- and inter-personal levels and impact on voice hearing experiences, that mirroring can occur between these two levels, and the role of power in relationships. Extending this last point regarding power, we previously made specific reference to the bullying nature of distressing voices as this tends to be the most troublesome dynamic for voice hearers to try and live with. However, voice hearing experiences can change over time and, contrary to popular belief, can greatly improve. In this chapter, we focus on voice profiling to help increase our understanding of this journey and subsequent relational experiences with voices.

Voice profiling: from chaos to order

The form of profiling we teach in our training workshops is influenced by the work of Coleman and Smith (1997) and the Maastricht Interview developed from the work of Marius Romme and Sandra Escher. It is commonly utilised by voice hearers and practitioners to explore possible links between voices and voice hearers' life experiences. The Maastricht Interview was pivotal in berthing a new understanding of voice hearing and challenges the biomedical explanation of voices and other unusual experiences such as visions. Voice profiling is delivered by many trainers across the world either as part of the Maastricht approach or a derivative of the original Maastricht Interview. There are some great examples of voice profiling literature available. For example, Coleman and Smith (1997) offer a workbook to explore the voice hearing experience and this includes a tabulated form of profiling.

We provide an example voice profile below of some of Ruth Lafferty (RL)'s voices (Table 6.1). We construct tabulated profiles similar to this during our training workshops. Following the voice profile, we discuss how we gather information to develop a voice profile and how this can be subsequently used by voice hearers to create greater understanding of their voices and relationships. As a warning, there are several profane words listed in the profile as direct quotations from voices. If

DOI: 10.4324/9781032619910-9

Table 6.1 Voice profile of a selection of RL's voices

Name and age	Gender	Other senses	Positive negative neutral	Command, advisory, commentary, soothing, insulting	Role	Examples of what voice says Voice tone
Grande 1st Voice RL heard 59 years	Male	Strong presence Often shadowy visual presence at my right shoulder	85% positive/ neutral Rarely negative now	Mostly advisory with commands now (Previously command and insulting)	"In Charge" "Guardian of the fence" Protector	"You stupid fucker" "Do this" "Don't do that" "Stupid" "Listen to ME" "Thank you", "That's the right thing", "Yes, I will talk with you" *Powerful Voice*
George (was **Georgia**) 59 years	Male (female until I was 19 years old)	None	Positive and neutral	Commentary, occasionally soothing and very occasionally advisory	Grande's 1st ally, Gentle Sage	"I think that's ok" "Perhaps listen to Grande" "Perhaps don't listen to Bill" *Meek Voice*
Little Ruth 5 years	Female	None	Negative on a "bad day" or neutral/ distressed	None	Indicator of distress, especially when I am "cut off" from my anxiety or distress.	Whimpering or sobbing occasionally, howling *Distressed Child*
Bill Late 60s yrs (until recently was fixed at 45 years)	Male	Visual Male, 11 feet tall. George recently noticed he is getting shorter	Negative	Command insulting	Intimidator (more likely indicator of stress if reminded of previous dangerous situations)	*Powerful Bellowing Voice*

(Continued)

Table 6.1 (Continued)

Name and age	Gender	Other senses	Positive negative neutral	Command, advisory, commentary, soothing, insulting	Role	Examples of what voice says / Voice tone
Honour (previously called The Misogynist by RL) 49 years	Male	Tactile: slapping and spitting	Negative, now moving to positive	Command insulting	"Oppressor" "Instructor"	"you fucking slut, whore, slag" "Curl up and die" "You need pegging out and flogging" "answer back", "defend yourself" *Loud Sneering Voice*
Courage (previously called 7th voice by RL) 38/9 years	Male	Tactile: pushing between shoulders	Negative, now moving to positive	Command and sometimes insulting (previously very insulting)	Pusher/instructor	"Fucking move", "fucking get going", "get out of my fucking way" *Gruff Voice*
D	Male	none	Negative/neutral (now silent, having stopped speaking after starting an art course)	Command, commentary		"Don't you get it, you idiot" "you get on my nerves" "why are you doing that"
Matrix 49 years	Male	Constant visual. Tall man in a long leather coat and leather hat. Neutral facial expression	Negative to neutral	Not verbal. Previously very irksome and sinister presence. Now irksome only when very close	Indicator of anxiety and threat of feeling exposed	Speaks through movement – is always visible. Moves closer, the more anxious I am. Difficult to negotiate with but sometimes now responds to polite "move further away" requests

Key: Names of Voices in bold – this is where voices have told RL their names as opposed to the names RL has given them.

profane words are difficult for you to read, please skip the column: "Examples of what the voice says" on the far right of the Profile table.

All of RL's voices discussed in the above profile were consulted at the time of writing and prior to going to publication. They all agreed to be described in this book. None of their agreements were obtained second hand by another voice. Where voices did not agree directly, voices were thanked and have not been included. The communication with Little Ruth is always difficult because she does not use words. RL explained the permission and the task and asked her to make a noise if she did not want this to happen. She was silent after each interaction, and so RL has taken this as her agreement to be included in this publication. RL had consulted Bill several times for permission to include the details about him. Each time he refused, but after there had been some changes in RL's relationship with Bill, he made no verbal response when asked for permission. RL concluded that it was safe to use information about him for the profile as he would currently not give a positive "yes", but not saying "no" felt like a sufficient level of agreement. RL's final decision to include the voices listed above was based on her own autonomous decision having respectfully consulted her voices and felt the final decision rested with her.

The structure of profiling, especially when approached with the assistance of a supportive other, may help you in several ways. It enables space between the experience of hearing voices and thinking about voices. This is important because, typically, we react to things we see, hear, etc., and this can often be influenced by our appraisal of the situation and associated emotions. This means that we don't always come to reliable conclusions. They are likely to be fuelled by our thoughts and how we are feeling at the time. Profiling also provides a space for voice hearers to step back and see a written recollection of their experience in a grid form that can invite reflection. As such, there is more emotional distance and space to reflect on the elements of personal experience and thus bring a sense of control or at least containment. Voice profiles are tangible records of experience that voice hearers can keep or share with a trusted other and can be something to come back to and think and/or talk about. They can also be developed and evolve gradually so that the process of disclosure is less overwhelming. As such, a voice profile can offer clues and points for thinking about possible links between the qualities of each voice and how they relate to personal experiences. Finally, they can also be a discussion point with a voice either in a talking-with-voices conversation or through mark-making (which we discuss in Chapter 8).

Completing a voice profile

Although this section in which we discuss how to profile voices is aimed at all readers, we especially wish to connect with those who hear voices.

The voice profile example we have provided above is intended to stimulate ideas for readers to help in their efforts to change voice hearing experiences. There is no magic here! Constructing a table in whichever way you find useful is the best way we have found to profile. This can include using separate sheets of paper for each section or each voice; drawing the information rather than using words, using coloured pens or pencils to signify different voices or qualities that are significant to each individual, adding drawings or diagrams or whatever fits with who you are. It is your information, and you can create whatever works best for you. How and where this information is kept can be very important for people who hear voices and to manage any sense of vulnerability that may be experienced, it is vital for the voice hearers to make these decisions.

Trying to get to know, organise, and live more peacefully with voices is not always a straightforward process and a few steps forward may trigger voices and your threat system because it's a move that may be slightly outside your comfort zone. It may also feel like a tremendous relief to find a way of sorting out so many elements of your voice hearing. In relation to the Tripartite Relationship Theory, this concerns doing something active to develop personal self-agency, improve the interpersonal dynamic, and contribute towards sense-making of voice hearing. This in turn can help you understand voice-related experiences and increase confidence in turning attention to voices rather than avoiding them. Turning curiously towards voices can be a critical step as avoidance of voices may maintain your anxiety about the power voices can have over you. Taking the process at a pace that allows progress without too much fatigue is individual to each person and each voice. Part of the process is being able to tolerate the uncertainty of whether a breakthrough can be made or whether it will feel tumultuous before settling again. In RL's experience, when there is a voice or voices that kick back, they are doing their job. RL interprets this as the voices trying to protect her and themselves. This might be true for readers and other voice hearers too.

Initially, voices may be suspicious of you doing something new that involves them. Try speaking to them in a reassuring way, confirming that you wish to get to know them better as you do this. Taking a step forward, in the case of profiling, filling in some of the grid with information about voices so you can stand back and look at it may feel exposing to voices. They do settle and accommodate so listening to them and your own anxiety is crucial so that you don't do too much and overwhelm yourself. A steady pace is the most progressive. Some voices are easier and almost eager to be identified and respectfully understood. You may know who these voices are already and that is a good place to start.

An example of making sense of voices through profiling: RL, Grande, and George

Profiling my voices helped me to explore who or what my voices are and where they come from. The more I have profiled my voices, the more sense I make of their role and have concluded them to be primarily protective. It's not always clear and it's usually paradoxical. As evident in the above voice profile, they often sound coercive, hostile and it feels like they are designed to annihilate dignity and self-agency. Anyone reading from the profile examples of what my voices say to me, and their aggressive tone, might consider it ridiculous that I postulate these transactions are protective.

However, as we have discussed in previous chapters, when voices are amenable to talking in a conversational way, and they take some time to trust and get used to talking in this way, I pick up clues that need decoding. For example, much of Grande's content concerned directives about obeying him, and how stupid, useless, and pointless I am. Through voice profiling, I questioned what examples such as these meant. I remember an occasion from my childhood when my father yelled at me, asking if I was stupid, why had I done such a stupid thing and not listened to him repeatedly and that I was to be sent to my room. I was about six years old and had a habit of getting excited if I saw something interesting on the other side of a road and would run towards the road. The hostile outburst with sanctions was because he was scared that I would get hit by a car, angry that I didn't seem to take in his warnings and had to be stopped by his anger rather than stopping myself and not frightening him! His level of energy – anger driven by terror – made me stop and not run into the road. He drew my attention to something dangerous that a sweet encouragement to stop and think would possibly fail with potentially damaging or fatal consequences. After my father calmed down and I had recovered from the shock of his energy, we chatted and hugged and I promised to think before running towards a road.

I initially felt what I now believe was shame for disappointing and scaring my father, but it had a profound effect on me and brought into my direct awareness how protective my father felt towards me and consequently how important my brother and I were to him. Many children and parents recognise this or similar scenarios. The memory of this event with my father came strongly to mind during times when I was curled up and trying to distance myself from what I felt was an unfair berating from Grande, whilst a number of other voices, triggered by Grande's escalating anger, were fighting amongst themselves. Voices do not usually initially explain directly why they are angry or hostile or what they want you to do differently. They don't seem to be open to negotiation immediately and usually they do not have a reassuring chat afterwards to make sure everyone is ok after anger is expressed, in the same way that my father did. However, it is possible to build understanding with a voice where directness and fairness become the marks of the relationship, such as my relationship with George. George is not only a voice that is strongly connected to some of my most difficult early experiences but is also the voice that has the mildest way of speaking. He is also becoming a stronger ally to Grande. When there is strong emotion and lively voices, I now seek out George's voice and energy as a starting point to then engage with more demanding voices.

Recalling memories such as this of my father's protective anger provided me with clues in my quest to discover the purpose of my voices. I started to think about the possibility of them also being protective. I was able to keep this in mind even during verbal assaults. When voices are speaking aggressively, it can be difficult to think clearly. This task of noticing and stepping back gave me both a way of giving me some distance from the strong emotional energy from my voices and also a way of getting close, to notice who they were and to try and understand them more. Thinking about their possible role gave me both useful distance and useful closeness which was the reverse of how I had previously responded. I had previously tried to distance myself from my voices, which exacerbated their frustration and made me more fearful of them and led to further distancing. Constructing meaning relating to the purpose and role of voices and their subsequent communications helped me to identify a context to their aggressive energy and not take it so personally. It helped me explore the reasons why they get distressed at me and ask them direct questions as well as informing my Talking with Voices communications with them (we will discuss this in more detail in Chapter 8). I have come to understand Grande and George as my primary protectors and others as pushers so that I do things that are good for me and help my well-being, which is also ultimately protective.

I am aware as I write this account that not everyone has experienced a parent or caregiver that was sufficiently loving and safe. I feel strongly that having a sense of the presence of someone that you experienced as safe and nurturing does something positive in helping to build a sense of safety and self-worth in the world and in yourself. I encourage anyone to spend some quiet, private time thinking about a person or people who have treated you well and what they were "saying" to you directly or indirectly in the way they treated you. For example, an aunt or grandparent or a teacher who looked out for you and wanted you to do well, enjoy your life, and be safe, despite also saying some tough things. A caring teacher may seem harshly tell you off and issue detentions but somehow you might know they have your back and want you to do well. The paradox of voices is that, because they may speak of the more difficult times in your life, they often speak harshly and seem to want to undermine the kind of safety related to your self-worth. Having a counter to these statements and reminding yourself of your own worth, having examples to call on when you are trying to interpret the intentions of your voice's current tirade may help you to distance and think about your voice and perhaps you can take their concern without taking the method of delivery so personally and so be able to make sense of the message.

I am also reminded of the potent example in Chapter 3 that Frank shared of the safe and nurturing garden space that he had built for himself and his voices. I cannot help but connect this with offering a relational kindness, self to self. His constructed garden seems to represent many things and one of them is developing a rich and supportive relationship with himself. A person he could rely on to look after him and take him to a safe place when trying to navigate difficult relationships and situations: Himself.

It could be argued because I developed a hunch that voices are protective, then I project this onto the way they speak to me. And that is true. We live through projection and construct our reality. This discovery has been pivotal in improving my relationships with my voices, and that is my truth, so I share it with you in case it may be useful to you too.

Useful steps to get started

1 If you decide to profile some or all of your voices, give yourself some good uninterrupted time if you are doing it alone, or preferably share the experience with a practitioner who has expressed interest, or a supportive friend or relative. Perhaps they would like to read sections of this book to help you both have a mutual understanding of profiling.
2 You can start completing the table however you wish. For example, begin by listing all your voices, or with one voice, and go across filling in the age you think they are, their gender, and so on.
3 If a voice has a name that you have given them, consider asking them if they have a name they call themselves. It may be different from the one you have given them and it may give you some clues as to what their role is and give them a sense of being included in the process. You may not want to do this for good reason, or not at this point, but it may be worth bearing in mind for your ongoing relationship building with a voice.
4 You can make notes of what voices say during the process if you feel this is helpful and even include the comments in the profile. If you find they are interrupting too much, try asking them to leave you to fill in the table so you have space to think. If they are suspicious and agitated and use commands or insults to try and stop you, try to reassure them that you are doing this so you can

understand them better. You know your voices best and what may work for you at this point. Remember, you can take as much time and as many pauses as you like.

5   Some parts of the profile might be more difficult to think about. Remember, there are no wrong answers. For example, a voice's "role" may need more thought than age or gender. It may take time to understand what their role is and they may have multiple roles which may change over time. These aspects often emerge over time the more you get to know and understand your voices.

6   If there is a voice that is particularly difficult for you to think about and you fear triggering them to become more distressing, it may be worth considering writing down some words or statements to clarify your good intent towards them. Writing things down can be powerful for you and your voices. It's rather like receiving an important letter and is a tangible record, almost a contract, between you and your voice.

7   If there are other things that are important to you that are not included in the voice profile table, add another heading. For example, it may be very important to you when certain voices are more lively or aggressive. You can add a heading such as "Most often upset by...".

8   When you have had enough for one session, remember to reward yourself and remind yourself that you are doing something helpful and courageous. Treat yourself!

As we grow and change over time, so too can our voices. A voice profile therefore can change and evolve over time. You can use it like a diary, revisiting it now and again but especially when experiencing significant change, and it can help you recognise your own growth and your reclaiming of power back into your life. This doesn't mean in a combative way that subjugates voices, but growing in your autonomy, freedom, and level of self-agency.

Concluding thoughts

Compartmentalising information about voices in a voice profile table can potentially create a false sense of simplicity. It is a construct but can feel like a reductionist process if the mindset to completing profiling is similar to simply filling out a form. Instead, the aim is to contribute to developing an understanding of any possible links between voices and life experiences, and this can become easier when some of the characteristics of voices are unpacked and documented. Voice hearers can experience a real benefit from disentangling voices and gaining an internal space to think about them, which is useful as an end point in itself. The extra value can be in using profiling to separate out these different voices and then to explore the links between voices and personal life story. This allows the deeper exploration of the links between voices and the past experiences that have left the wounds that voices point to. It is a cyclical process of deconstructing aspects of voices to reconstruct an understanding of them in a new and more sophisticated way that makes who voices are more apparent to the voice hearer and helps the voice hearer discover who voices are and why they are with them.

Practitioners and supporters who are informed by the Tripartite Relationship Theory can play a role in supporting a voice hearer to explore their voices through profiling. Being alongside and having compassion and support in the room whilst undertaking what may feel like a challenging process may help a voice hearer make profound changes in their lives and with their voices.

Chapter 7

Mapping

Life and voices

We explained in Chapter 6 that we consider voice profiling, voice mapping, and communicating with voices as being interlinked. For the purpose of the book, we describe these as separate, distinct activities, but in real-world practice, we advocate for a flexible and integrative approach, wherein profiling, mapping, and communicating inform each other. These three activities ought to be considered collectively a means of acquiring knowledge, informing understanding, and facilitating communication with voices. Although we don't consider there to be a prescribed starting point, in Chapter 6, we discussed the process and value of voice profiling and one of us (RL) shared examples of their own voice profiling work relating to their voices. In this chapter, we discuss our approach to mapping lives and voices. In Chapter 8, we will discuss communicating with voices.

Mapping lives

In the opening two chapters of this book, we stated our belief that voice hearing experiences for many people are rooted in the life histories of voice hearers, and it is for voice hearers themselves to construct their own personal meaning associated with their voices through investigating their own historical clues. It can be helpful, therefore, to map voice hearers' unique life histories. Although we don't prescribe a fixed way for a person to map their life, a common element to this activity is the telling of life stories through a diagrammatic representation on paper of various milestones across the stages of voice hearers' lives, from the earliest points they can remember to the present date. Some people prefer to draw a linear line across a piece of paper (or flip chart) from their earliest recollections to their most recent, with various points identified between these two ends where they have recalled significant events. Others prefer to be more creative and include, for example, symbols to represent places or events, or perhaps use metaphors such as a river to represent their flow of life, or perhaps even use different colours to emphasise different mood states. There are numerous ways to draw one's own life map (see Figure 7.1). Common to all these different ways, the aim is for voice hearers to identify points in their lives they consider significant and to reflect on what happened at that time in their life to help reconstruct the context from their various

DOI: 10.4324/9781032619910-10

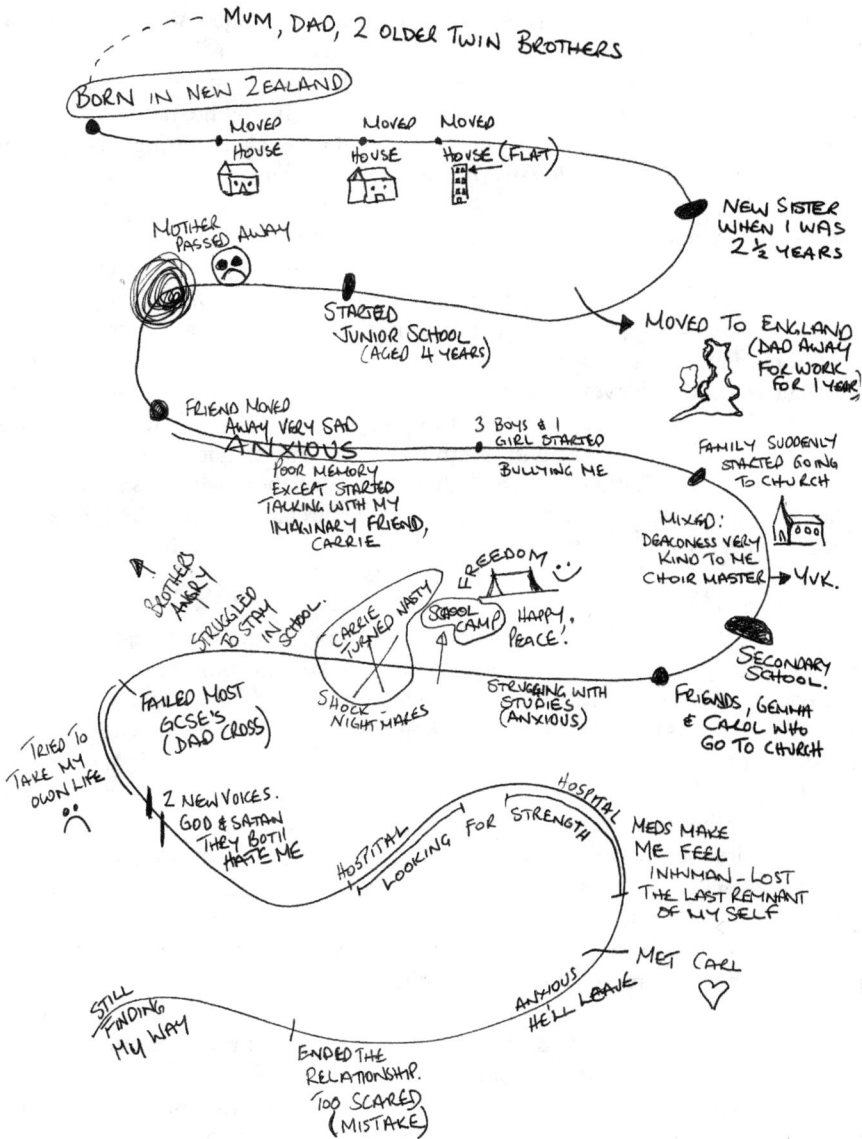

MUM, DAD, 2 OLDER TWIN BROTHERS

BORN IN NEW ZEALAND

MOVED HOUSE

MOVED HOUSE

MOVED HOUSE (FLAT)

NEW SISTER WHEN I WAS 2½ YEARS

MOTHER PASSED AWAY

STARTED JUNIOR SCHOOL (AGED 4 YEARS)

MOVED TO ENGLAND (DAD AWAY FOR WORK FOR 1 YEAR)

FRIEND MOVED AWAY VERY SAD
ANXIOUS

3 BOYS & 1 GIRL STARTED

POOR MEMORY EXCEPT STARTED TALKING WITH MY IMAGINARY FRIEND, CARRIE

BULLYING ME

FAMILY SUDDENLY STARTED GOING TO CHURCH

MIXED: DEACONESS VERY KIND TO ME CHOIR MASTER → YVK.

BROTHER ANGRY

STRUGGLED TO STAY IN SCHOOL

CARRIE TURNED NASTY

FREEDOM

SCHOOL CAMP

HAPPY, PEACE!

FAILED MOST GCSE's (DAD CROSS)

SHOCK NIGHTMARES

STRUGGLING WITH STUDIES (ANXIOUS)

SECONDARY SCHOOL.

FRIENDS, GEMMA & CAROL WHO GO TO CHURCH

TRIED TO TAKE MY OWN LIFE

2 NEW VOICES. GOD & SATAN THEY BOTH HATE ME

HOSPITAL

LOOKING FOR STRENGTH

HOSPITAL

MEDS MAKE ME FEEL INHUMAN - LOST THE LAST REMNANT OF MYSELF

MET CARL ♡

STILL FINDING MY WAY

ENDED THE RELATIONSHIP. TOO SCARED (MISTAKE)

ANXIOUS HE'LL LEAVE

Figure 7.1 Example of a life map.

points in their life, i.e., who was involved, what they and others were doing at that time, and what emotions and thoughts they can recall from that time. When all the events have been recalled and recorded on their life map, we then ask voice hearers to go through it again to see if they can identify any themes. There might be any number of themes, for example, some might include recurring examples of loneliness or isolation or feeling overpowered to name but a few. We also ask voice hearers, if they hadn't already done so, to identify on their life map when they first began to hear voices and any subsequent voices thereafter.

It is important to keep in mind that the person completing the exercise should remain in control of how much information they disclose (and when) and how they want to record it on their life map. Respecting and supporting voice hearers to assert their boundaries when completing this exercise is an important contribution to enhance their own "level of agency". For example, asserting oneself interperson- ally can help with the development of assertion intra-personally with voices. This is an important issue that we will return to later in this chapter when we discuss voice mapping. In addition to a person learning more about what has happened at various points during their life, details relating to circumstances around the emer- gence of voice(s), and how they have responded to any adverse difficulties, there is also an overarching aim during the life mapping process to build a sense of agency and construct personal meaning.

Given the above consideration regarding disclosure, in our experience, complet- ing a life map typically happens in layers and can take some time. It can be difficult for any of us to recall and record events from the past. Not only can it require effort to search for events deep in our memories but, especially for anyone with upsetting memories from past events, it can feel traumatic. For some people in these situa- tions, their effort might have been spent pushing away memories into the back of their minds rather than recalling them. So, to ask someone to investigate their life history requires sensitivity. As such, usually a person initially records on their life map a range of events about which feel less emotionally loaded and less distressing by others knowing. Often, especially if the person is working closely with a part- ner (i.e., another workshop participant or, away from the workshop, a person they trust), they may feel more comfortable going through their life map for a second time to record more events and/or add more detail to previously recorded events. This layered approach might continue and would include revisiting the life map several times and over a long period.

The learning from recording a life map, even when incomplete, can inform the voice profile discussed in Chapter 6, help add meaning to the voice mapping exercise (discussed below), and inform communication with voices (discussed in Chapter 8). To repeat our earlier point, this is a reciprocal process.

Mapping voices: applying the Voice Dialogue method

In addition to completing a life map to learn and understand more about voices, we also advocate completing a voice map. Again, these should be considered integrated: each informs the other. Before we discuss how we typically map a person's voices, we want to first acknowledge the Voice Dialogue approach of Stone and Stone (1989) (also see our previous work, Lafferty & Allison (2021), for a discussion regarding our application of this). Briefly, Voice Dialogue is an approach rooted in psychodynamic theory and aimed at exploring relational difficulties with oneself and others. According to Stone and Stone, rather than having single consistent identities, we are all comprised of multiple "selves" (they use this and several other terms interchangeably: sub-personalities, parts, energies), some of which Stone and Stone refer to as primary, and some they refer to as disowned that help us to manage our daily social interactions. The primary selves are more noticeable in their influence on how we manage social situations. For example, one of our selves may be known to us as a "pleaser", which dominates when we try to please other people all the time; or we may know another one of our dominant selves as a "critic", recognisable when we criticise ourselves or others. By contrast, the disowned selves are those which we have learned might be socially undesirable or have attributes we don't like and, consequently, we have pushed away. For example, we might have recognised one of our selves as "selfish", which is typically less appealing to others than, say, a pleaser and so we might have disowned this part of ourselves. According to Stone and Stone, this disowning is problematic in that the disowned "selfish" part, for example, can operate unconsciously in our lives. It can also serve an important function for the individual concerned, which has been negated through the disowning. For example, without embracing (to some extent) a "selfish" part, one's own well-being and self-care needs are disregarded and unmet. Stone and Stone construct what they refer to as a psychic map (see Figure 7.2) to represent these different parts/selves, which enables the individual concerned to differentiate, understand, and communicate with their different selves. It also enables the individual to identify where their different "selves" are in relation to oneself, i.e., which "selves" are closer and perhaps more active in their lives and which ones are perhaps less involved, or even ignored or pushed away.

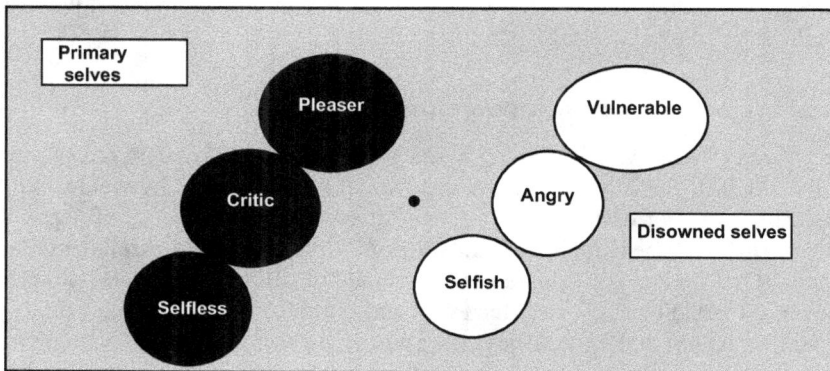

Figure 7.2 Stone and Stone's psychic map.

Importantly for voice hearing, Voice Dialogue theory has been usefully applied in the work of the Hearing Voices Movement to communication processes with voices. This has been in recognition of a close alignment of the principles of learning to understand and communicate with different selves or voices. This adaptation, wherein the emphasis is on voices rather than selves, has seen the approach re-named in the voice hearing community as "Talking with Voices". We discuss this in more detail in Chapter 8 but, for now, we illustrate below how we apply Stone and Stone's psychic map to voices rather than selves.

Why map voices?

Mapping voices might, at first, seem unusual. In principle, it is similar to the psychic map described above but, instead of different "selves", voices are mapped in relation to the voice hearer. This can be documented on paper but, several years ago, we began to experiment with an idea to make voice mapping more dynamic and interactive for voice hearers and to enable workshop participants to benefit from observing or taking part. Undertaking a voice mapping exercise might first feel challenging but, importantly, we have found it to be empowering for voice hearers (and, in some cases, their voices). Through completing a voice map, a voice hearer reconstructs a representation of the location of their voices in relation to themselves. Doing so enables an examination and appreciation of dynamic relations between a voice hearer and their voices, and also between the different voices. It also enables opportunities to explore potential contributory factors to voice hearing experiences and potential ways to change voice hearing experiences.

In the following section, we share an activity we normally undertake during our voice hearing workshops to illustrate how relational dynamics previously discussed in this and earlier chapters play out and can be experienced by a person hearing voices. To aid the discussion about the activity, we focus on one of us as a voice hearer (Ruth Lafferty (RL)) and one of us as a facilitator (Rob Allison (RA)). The aim is to physically map RL's voices and develop a helpful understanding of the relational context between RL and her voices and amongst her voices. We structure the activity into two stages, discussed below.

Mapping voices activity: stage one

We typically begin with RL taking a seat in the centre of the room (represented by the small dot in Figure 7.3) and confirming which voices she would like to map. The names of each voice are then written on separate pieces of paper. To illustrate the exercise here, we include nine of RL's voices (in no particular order): Grande (Gr), George (G), Honour (H), Courage (C) Bill (B), the three watchers (Matrix [M] and the Clipboard Men [W]), and Little Ruth (R) (see Figure 7.3).

Once the names of the voices have been written on pieces of paper, RL nominates workshop participants to represent each of her voices until all the voices have been allocated. During this process, we encourage participants to avoid personalising

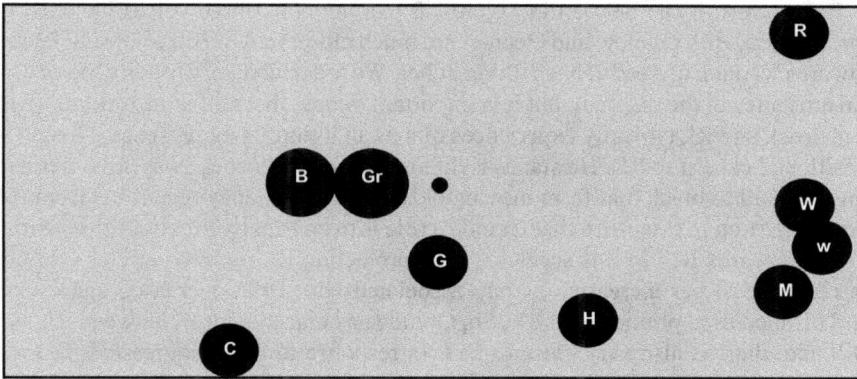

Figure 7.3 Mapping of RL's voices.

their allocation, i.e., the intention is to offer everyone an opportunity to take part in the exercise rather than match a particular voice to a particular participant. Following this, RL identifies whereabouts in the room she would like the nominated participant to move towards to represent where she locates her voice in real time and space. This continues until all the participants have moved to their respective points in the room, illustrated in Figure 7.3.

Participants' positions in their allocated places might involve them standing, sitting, or laying down; they may be very close to RL or far away (within the confines of the room); they may be facing towards RL or away from her or towards a wall, or facing towards another participant representing a different voice. These various positions depend on different voices; each voice typically occupies a different position in the room. RL also typically states whether the voices remain static or move around but, for the purpose of this first stage of the exercise, they are typically static (we will explain shortly, during the second stage of the exercise, how we facilitate the movement of voices).

Each time a participant is asked to move to a specific point in the room with their allocated voice, we discuss the reason for this specific location and what the voice is doing (or would typically do) at that moment. For example, Little Ruth is usually located at the furthest corner of the room, sitting on the floor, and facing towards the corner. She is almost always in a corner or generally furthest away and usually upset and very quiet. The three watchers are also far from RL but towards the centre of the wall. They are always visible. They stand quietly, watching RL and the activities taking place around her. They typically move closer if RL's stress levels increase, so RL identifies a direct correlation between her emotional state and their proximity. Honour and Courage are slightly closer and have a connection to each other. If one of them moves or shows strong oppressive energy, the shift typically engages the other and they either "work together" or they become combative with each other and possibly other voices, such as Grande.

By contrast, it can be seen in Figure 7.3 that the other three voices included in the exercise, Bill, Grande, and George, are much closer to RL. Bill is closely facing towards RL and aggressively shouting at her. We are unable to represent the physical attributes in the diagram, but it is important to note that Bill is 11 feet tall (over 3 metres), and RL typically experiences him as an intimidating presence. Grande is positioned closest to RL. He stands right next to her but facing away from her and towards Bill to block him from moving closer to RL. You may remember from the voice profiling in Chapter 6 that Grande's role is to constantly monitor for potential threats towards RL. In this scenario, he is protecting RL by moving closer to her in response to her increased anxiety associated with Bill's increased aggression and his increased proximity to RL. So, Grande has placed himself between RL and Bill and, thus, is also very close to Bill. In response to Bill's aggression, Grande is also shouting back at him. George is located in a similar proximity to RL as Bill but is directly in front of RL. Again, referring to the voice profile in Chapter 6, you may remember that George is an ally to Grande. As such, he is trying to support Grande, and in turn RL, in the current situation.

One of the most immediate responses usually evoked in the group at this stage is recognition of the intensity of the situation for RL. The interaction between Grande and Bill is reported by RL as loud, hostile, and taking place almost on top of her, leaving very little space for self. For RL, this can feel overwhelming and distracting, which usually makes it difficult for her to engage with other people at that moment and, consequently, she works hard to focus on the present and her surroundings to help her engage interpersonally with others. Through physically mapping voices in this way, other group participants can see how close these voice interactions take place around RL. We can also increase an appreciation of this scenario by asking participants representing these three voices, for example, to talk out loud at a similar volume to the voices. This enhances an appreciation of the overall intensity of the situation for RL. The first stage of the exercise is complete when all the voices, represented by the workshop participants, have been placed at their respective points in the room.

This can be a helpful learning opportunity in that it physically illustrates where voices are located and enables a shared understanding and empathy regarding a voice hearing experience, in this case for RL. If you are curious enough, we recommend you give this activity a try. However, we appreciate that it can be difficult to replicate, especially if you do not have other people to take part. If you do have someone (or maybe a few people) with whom you feel comfortable enough to trust and share this activity, then we encourage you to work together and try this. If this is possible for you, then great. If this is not possible for you, then we believe that there is a lot of benefit to be gained from thinking and reflecting on how this applies to you as you read about this activity. You could replicate this exercise by using buttons on a table or using furniture to represent different voices. If you feel comfortable enough to reflect on this, then we encourage you to put some time aside, perhaps gather a pen and some paper if you find it helpful to jot things down for your recollection, and to consider how the questions we discuss in the next stage below might relate to you and your voices.

Some of you may be surprised to learn that voices are not static. They have an energy, which can change, and they can move around in relation to the voice hearer and to other voices (as we describe in this scenario). We try to capture this dynamic shifting of energy in the second stage of the activity, which builds on the first stage and provides a more powerful learning opportunity in that we explore how to change the voice hearing experience by moving the position of voices and influencing their energies. In doing so, the second stage expands on the static representation of voices in the first stage and explores in more detail the shifting energies amongst voices, to understand the circumstances in which this happens, and the consequences of this.

Mapping voices activity: stage two

The line of questioning when facilitating the second stage unfolds in one of two ways (although the process we undertake to facilitate this is the same). This depends on whether the mapping constructed in the first stage (i.e., Figure 7.3) represented either the usual position of voices (to aid our description of this here, we will call this option "a") or whether it represented something more atypical (option "b"), for example, if the voice hearer was feeling more distressed than usual and, associated with this, their voices had changed from their usual positions. For either of the two options, the broad aim is to help reduce levels of distress felt by the voice hearer by exploring how they can move their voices regardless of whether the voices are currently in their usual (option "a") or unusual (option "b") positions. If the voices are in their usual positions (option "a"), then we undertake a line of questioning aimed at helping the voice hearer consider how they would prefer to experience their voice(s) and how they might move their voice(s) to a new position to reflect this preferred experience. If the voices are not in their usual position but instead in a different position (option "b"), then we would undertake a line of questioning aimed at helping the voice hearer explore what might have influenced this change and how they might move the voice(s) back to their usual (or possibly a new) position to help reduce the voice hearer's level of distress. The difference between the two options concerns whether we explore new positions or how to return to more stable positions. Regardless, the process is the same for either option.

Returning to RL's scenario, we typically begin the second stage with RL confirming whether her voice map from the first stage typically represented the position and energy levels of her voices. In the example we have described above, most voices were positioned where they would usually be in relation to RL apart from Bill, Grande, and George. During less stressful times for RL, these three voices are usually positioned further away from her and, consequently, she would have felt more space around her, which she associates with feeling less stressed. Figure 7.4 illustrates where these three voices would usually be in relation to RL. As illustrated, Bill would be further away from RL to her right-hand side, remaining just in her eyeline. Grande would also usually be slightly further away from RL but in front of her. So too for George, who would also usually be slightly further away from RL and in front of her. So, the aim for RL in this activity was to understand

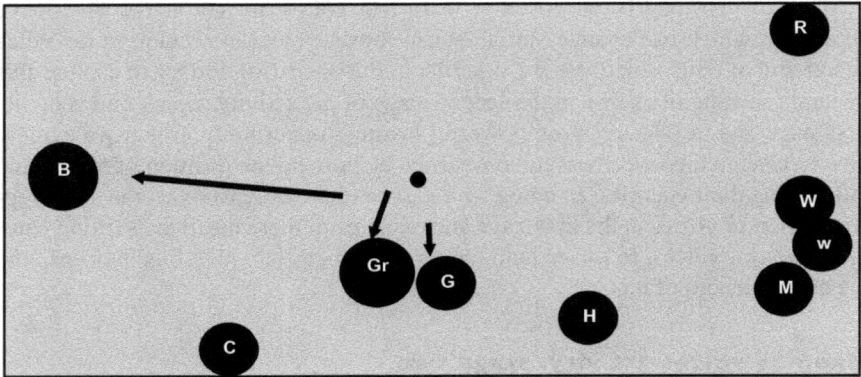

Figure 7.4 Moving RL's voices to their usual positions.

why these three voices had moved closer than usual to her and then, at least initially, to facilitate them moving back to their usual positions.

Establishing these details can provide an empowering opportunity for a person distressed by voice hearing. It can provide them space to reflect on what might have happened intra-personally (i.e., the relational context between the voice hearer and their voices) to have influenced their energy levels, and the position of voices in relation to the voice hearer, and what might have happened inter-personally with other people (i.e., the relational context between the voice hearer and their external world) to have influenced this. In other words, it reinforces the notion that voices, and voice hearing, happen not in isolation but in the context of a voice hearer's life and, as such, provides an opportunity to consider how events happening in one's own life might contribute to their voice's activity and subsequent voice hearing experience.

Voice mapping to change voice hearing experiences

Reaching this point in the activity enables an opportunity to explore an important question: how might voice hearing experiences be changed? In our discussion about this, by referring to RL's specific scenario to pose specific questions and illustrate key points, we hope that this encourages you to consider how these questions might apply to you and your situation.

Before you think about a similar question for you and your voices, however, we would like to give you two pieces of advice based on our experience of trying to make this an effective activity. First, try to focus on one voice at a time. RL began with Bill because she believed that this voice was the root of her distress at that time which stimulated a reaction from other voices. So, focusing on improving her overall voice hearing experience through first changing Bill's position and energy made sense to RL. We encourage you to similarly first select a voice that makes sense to you. Second, try to be patient with yourself and your voices as you complete the activity. For example, understandably, you may want one of your voices to move further away from you but immediately feel defeated because the voice won't move (and you may not know how to move the voice). This activity takes practice to develop competence and confidence. It would be unrealistic to expect anyone to try this for the first time, or even first several times, without struggling. For RL, knowing where she wanted Bill to move, and even willing him to move, did not mean that Bill immediately moved. This needed to be explored and carefully considered in relation to intra- and inter-personal contexts, which we discuss in more detail shortly.

Why voices move?

Returning to RL's scenario, another question we might ask is: what has happened in order for Bill, Grande, and George to have moved from their usual positions? As we have referred to numerous times throughout this book, and illustrated through the Tripartite Relationship Theory, events taking place in our inter-personal life influence events in our intra-personal life, and vice-versa. So, a starting point to answer this question is to reflect on recent and current interpersonal and intra-personal interactions. At first, the two may seem unconnected. However, we encourage you to mentally note or jot down on paper all the events that have happened over approximately the past month. This includes the people you have spent time with, talked to, and how conversations unfolded and what they were about. In doing this, it is important to also recall how you felt at that time, what was going through your mind at that time, and how you responded in those situations. For RL, there were events taking place in her interpersonal life context which led to her feeling conflicted and distressed. In trying to be supportive to others, her doing for others (i.e., her selflessness) became more dominant than doing for self (i.e., her selfishness) and, consequently, RL reflected that she had sacrificed too much of her own needs and became vulnerable. As this happened, and as we have seen illustrated in the voice mapping, RL's voice activity increased and they became more agitated, especially the energy levels of Bill, Grande, and George. Bill had moved aggressively closer to RL, Grande moved closer to protect RL, and George moved closer to support Grande and RL.

You may remember the "who's making sense?" theme from the Tripartite Relationship Theory, about which we stated the importance of not only making sense of voice hearing but also considering what influences this sense-making. We encourage you to become an expert in your own experience by exploring what has led you to hear voices and what has happened in your current situation to influence your voices. Sometimes it may not be obvious why voices say certain things and in a certain way. But, if you can give your time to search, you may find important clues. This can be important because there may be a pattern for a specific voice, wherein the voice responds to particular issues in your life. Exploring and finding meaning related to this can help you to develop an understanding of the way in which a voice reacts and can provide you with critical information that may help in your communication with that voice (we explore how to do this in Chapter 8) and explore whether there are things you want to change regarding how you relate to yourself, your voices, and other people. As well as making sense, small changes can increase self-agency, confidence, and resilience in the face of difficult voice interactions and may help when exploring ways to move a voice and, hence, change voice hearing experiences.

Where to move voices?

After we have considered what has happened, we ask another specific question: where would you like to move your voice(s) to help you feel less distressed/more comfortable? Sometimes, the response of a person distressed by their voices to this question might be to wish the voices would permanently go away. We can appreciate why someone might wish this. You may remember the work of Romme and Escher and several others we referred to earlier in this book. They pioneered for voice hearing to be conceptualised as providing historical links to the voice hearer's past, of which there is potential value, and without which their vulnerability might expose them to risky situations. For RL, making sense of this helped her to make sense of the current scenario we have illustrated here and provided her with an opportunity to take some control of an experience that she previously considered uncontrollable. RL wanted Bill to move back to the further distanced position he typically occupied, which aligned with a relatively calmer energy compared to the current overwhelming aggressive and threatening position he was occupying. You may similarly want one of your voices (remember, we suggest you only focus on one voice for now) to move to a further point from you, perhaps to where they would usually be or, if that is too difficult to imagine, to at least a less threatening place.

Moving voices to change voice hearing experiences

The final part of the activity involves exploring what is likely to be the most pressing question for readers of this book: how we can move voices and change voice hearing experiences? Returning to RL's scenario, we consider this with another specific question: what needs to happen to move Bill back again to his more distanced position and be experienced as less aggressive or threatening towards RL? Again, although we focus on RL's scenario here to help illustrate how we have approached this question, we encourage you to consider how you might approach a similar question related to your situation.

It is important to remember a key point we made at the beginning of this chapter: to get the most benefit from mapping voices, we recommend you consider it as part of an integrative approach involving voice profiling and communicating with voices (we describe communicating with voices in Chapter 8) to enable increased potential to influence voice hearing experiences. There are several reasons for this.

First, and to state what might seem obvious, just because a person may wish their voices would change (for example, by moving further away) does not mean change will automatically happen. This is the same for all of us in our relationships with other people, i.e., just because we may want a family member, friend, work colleague, etc. to change or do something specific, does not mean they will do it. In fact, in some cases, we may wish or even insist on this so much, but they become even more reluctant to do it! We can relate this to the "level of agency" theme of the Tripartite Relationship Theory. We believe that developing influence over one's voice hearing experience is, arguably, most important to voice hearers and essential to changing these experiences for the better. In RL's scenario, she has had to develop sufficient agency to assertively approach her voices in a respect-ful way and reclaim her own space by facilitating them to move (we explain how shortly). Asserting oneself is more than asking. A problem with asking is that it can be treated like a request and declined by voices. As such, it is helpful to under-stand effective ways of approaching and communicating with voices, which may differ between voice hearers and different voices. The voice profile discussed in Chapter 6 is a great way of collating information about voices that can inform the voice mapping exercise. This can also inform how we might "talk with voices" (explored in Chapter 8), which in turn can influence voice hearing experiences.

Second, to support the development of one's own sense of agency and subsequent understanding of ways to approach and communicate with voices, it is helpful to recall the "who's making sense?" theme of the Tripartite Relationship. As we rec-ollected above, more than simply understanding voices, it concerns awareness of how conventional understandings influence one's own voice hearing experiences and construction of a personally meaningful explanation of voice hearing. Again, compil-ing a voice profile (Chapter 6) and communicating with voices (Chapter 8) can help explore and collate information relevant to this. This can help voice hearers under-stand who their voices are, where they come from, and begin to consider how they might approach them in a voice mapping scenario perhaps similar to RL's.

Third, and again referring to the intra- and inter-personal connection, it is impor-tant to keep in mind that voice hearing experiences are influenced by what is hap-pening in the hearer's internal and external life contexts. In other words, attempts to make changes to the internal context (voices) are most effective when they take place alongside changes in the external context. Applying this notion to RL's voice mapping activity, we could pose a further question to ask of RL: "in order for Bill to be further away, what do you notice about yourself and your situation that would be different"? Asking a question such as this is aimed at encouraging reflection regarding the circumstances in which distressing voice-related experiences might be different from times when voices feel more settled. RL had recognised that some of her voices had changed and became increasingly aggressive and agitated at a time of changes to an inter-personal situation in her life with another person. Bill had become more abusive, insulting, energetic, and had moved more threateningly closer to RL, at a time when personal boundaries in an inter-personal relationship had been challenged and breached. Through constructing a personally meaningful explanation, RL concluded that her voices were reacting and feeling threatened by this inter-personal situation. RL interpreted this as a need for her to make changes to the inter-personal situation to help her make changes to her intra-personal experiences with her voices. In other words, and to answer the question concerning how RL could change her voice hearing experience, she concluded that she had to first make changes to the ways in which she related to either a specific person or people generally (i.e., her inter-personal life context).

Exploring the energy and movement of voices in this way through asking questions and encouraging reflection enables an empowering learning opportunity for a person to understand contextual influences on their voice hearing experience. This also suggests that voices can be considered a way of alarming voice hearers to issues in their life that need addressing. Constructing personal meaning can be an empowering process but requires the individual concerned to be clear regarding their self-responsibility to address any required changes, both intra- and inter-personally.

Finally, and fundamentally, we consider voice mapping to be a learning exercise. Extending the above points, and to reiterate our position set out at the beginning of the book, people who hear voices can share common experiences with other voice hearers but also have personally unique and meaningful experiences. There is no single approach that can benefit everyone to understand or change voice hearing experiences. As such, there is no generic question to ask or action to take, including those related to this voice mapping activity, that will be universally helpful to everyone. For this reason, although we have illustrated examples where RL's voice hearing experiences have changed and improved, we encourage you to explore how your own life circumstances might influence voice hearing and how you might apply this to benefit your voice hearing experience. Expanding on this point, if voice mapping is practiced in a safe and trusting setting, it offers an opportunity to try something that might ordinarily be perceived as unachievable. We encourage you to go into the activity with curiosity and an open mind. Rather than expect great and immediate changes, instead explore what you can learn from taking part and consider how this can help you and your experiences of your voices.

After confirming where voices might move to, there is then an opportunity to explore how a voice hearer might gain some influence over voices. Following consideration of the above points, RL was unable to move Bill during the voice mapping activity. Having reflected on her broader context discussed above, she had concluded that she needed to address and make changes to an inter-personal relationship as part of her efforts to change voice hearing experiences generally and her experience of Bill specifically. However, the mapping activity provided RL with an opportunity to explore further the movement of Bill. RL asked the nominated group participant representing Bill to walk over to the point in the room where Bill would ordinarily be. As previously stated, this would usually be further from RL, on her right-hand side, near the wall and just within her eyeline (see Figure 7.4). Asking a group participant to physically move to represent where RL would like Bill to be positioned enabled her an opportunity to reflect on how she might do this for herself and on her immediate thoughts and emotions related to this. This is an important step in the process. It illustrates dynamically to the self and the related voices, a position of intent, a plan, and a goal. It's a deliberate point in time that says, "I am going to make this happen". It is the engaging of an assertive energy.

We typically paused for a few minutes to encourage RL to gather her thoughts on Bill's new position and share her feelings about this. Questions are posed such as "now that Bill has moved further away, what is going through your mind right now"? and "how do you feel when you see Bill has moved further away"? It also provides an opportunity to explore how the movement of one voice impacts on other voices. For example, "what typically happens with other voices when Bill moves further away"? For RL, other voices would typically be less agitated and, more specifically, Grande would move a little further away from RL and centrally in front of her. Following Grande's movement, George would typically then also move slightly further away from RL.

Developing empathy with voices: exchanging positions

Mapping voices in this way also provides interesting opportunities for voice hearers to stand in the position occupied by voices, i.e., to effectively swap places with their voices. Doing so enables a person to view and reflect on their own scenario but from a different perspective and to consider the position taken up by their selected voice. During our illustrated voice mapping exercise, RL stood up from her chair and swapped places with the group participant representing Grande. This enabled her to see and think about her situation from a changed position and to also consider what it might be like for Grande, i.e., explore his view regarding other voices and especially his stance between RL and Bill and threats for Grande associated with this. For RL, this also provided a shift in emotion, to the extent that she became more accepting and compassionate towards Grande, and a shift in thinking in terms of reflecting on the responsibilities and subsequent actions she needed to take in her inter-personal relationships to bring about change to her voice hearing.

RL shares her recollection of constructing her voice map in Table 7.1. This is shared here to provide readers with some insight regarding the emotional impact of

Table 7.1 RL's reflections on the voice mapping activity

This exercise makes the invisible dynamic world of the voice hearer much more apparent. For me, the power of this exercise lies partly in the constructing of the scenario with time to think about various voices and my relationships with them from a slight distance. The exercise enables me to take a meta-position: observing the space in the room, voices, and self rather than being entirely immersed in the moment with the dynamic sensations of voices. Because my attention shifts to the people representing my voices, as well as the voices still being present in the room, this process does something paradoxical in giving both an opportunity to be more curious and make a stronger connection to voices. I can get closer to what voices are communicating and also create some distance to be able to think and feel at the same time. Creating distance in order to create connection, if you like. So, in order to get the most out of the learning experience, it is important to be as engaged as possible with the exercise and take time to construct it.

Engaging with this exercise can be graded, from thinking about it purposefully by making notes either with a trusted other or alone, then exploring the different stages of mapping a little at a time and seeing what insights emerge. Gradual engagement can build confidence in the process for both the voice hearer and their voices. The insights that emerge can build a sense of purpose and value, as well as helping me to make sense and find some agency with my voices.

(Continued)

Table 7.1 (Continued)

When we set up the exercise as we have described in this chapter, Bill had been moving about during the day and was more agitated than usual. Whilst this may have been related to the workshop and the number of people in the room, my experience of facilitating workshops and specifically the mapping exercise doesn't generally provoke this response from Bill. Typically, if Bill moves towards me aggressively, a number of other voices and myself react. Grande moves into a defensive position and becomes more verbal, louder, and highly assertive or even aggressive to counter Bill's energy. George moves closer to Grande to underline his allegiance to Grande's position and other voices become agitated, expressing and amplifying my own emotional responses to Bill: anxiety, some anger, and shame-related distress at the things Bill was saying. He was sneering, laughing, and insulting, repeating some familiar lines and scenarios. Grande was shouting at him and telling him to shut up and back away, attempting to assert authority and, on reflection, modelling this assertiveness to me.

The group exercise included asking the participant representing Bill to move to where I would prefer Bill to be standing. This juxtaposition of "what is" and "what I would prefer" helps me focus my attention on where I would like Bill to move to. It stands for hope that I can change things. It offered me a point to focus on when the room was full of noise and movement. As many voice hearers can probably identify, it is easy to get overwhelmed by a complex of strong emotion, such as anxiety, fear, disgust, and anger, when voices are increasingly distressed and start moving in atypical ways. It's difficult to think clearly and to act assertively and protectively. The dynamic reenactment of this scenario of feeling overwhelmed and unable to protect self is often a repeated theme from past experiences that may be linked to the emergence of my voices. The option of having someone representing a voice stand in a place where I would prefer that voice to be permitted my own attention and intention to move towards that point and moved me out of the habitual overwhelm and "stuckness", in which I felt I had to accept the position that Bill takes with me, accept or tolerate the berating, and, at best, allow Grande to "do the assertiveness for me". Whilst I accept that Grande is a part of me, I can argue that I am being assertive with Bill by Grande challenging him, but it is indirect, and "I" am not being assertive and using my own wilful self-agency directly for myself.

The insight I gained from this exercise was powerfully reinforced when I swapped places with the participant who represented Grande. I immediately felt the weight of responsibility to manage Bill and my protection. I felt tremendous empathy for the constant vigilance and his relentless advocacy for my safety and autonomy. I felt a tremendous love for Grande, and for George who I recognise as his ally. I couldn't make the connection that I was experiencing love and honouring for a part of myself. I understand this in theory, and I am trying to accept that this is an approximation of self-respect and self-worth. I can see that Grande is worthy of love, respect, and dignity. I could also see that he was entitled to a rest! This helped me to think about what he (or I) needed and that this included me being more directly assertive not only to Bill but within situations and relationships in my life where I don't use self-agency and don't set boundaries aligned with my own rights.

(Continued)

Table 7.1 (Continued)

These are the situations that trigger my voices to react most aggressively. The voices and emotional distress can either overwhelm me and I get cross with them, or I can see them for what they are: amplifiers of my own disowned distress, disowned rights, and disowned agency to identify and then hold good boundaries.

This exercise enabled me to see past the dynamic movement of voices and what they said and shouted in the room and offered me a stark enactment of the very dynamic that causes me so much intrapsychic distress and interpersonal anxiety. Finding ways of protecting myself from real and, more often, perceived interpersonal threat is the core of the dynamic that was illustrated in the voice mapping exercise.

The pathway to re-owning rights and seeing oneself as equally entitled to dignity and fair treatment from others and from oneself is a complex and difficult one. For me, developing assertiveness is part of that path, but I do not see assertiveness as learning a set of social skills and I would suggest that it is more than that for most people, including voice hearers. One of the issues that maintains the conflict with my voices and therefore myself is related to shame. A very complex, elusive, and deeply ingrained emotional experience that attaches to deeply personal experiences that are difficult to identify, talk about, and separate out. Exploring the role of shame in my own voice hearing and how it modulates capacity to be assertive has been demanding and difficult. It is an unfinished piece of explorative work, in terms of how it relates to the phenomena of voice hearing but one that I will return to at a later date.

The voice mapping exercise can offer an opportunity to explore the specific issue that a voice hearer regularly has to grapple with and being able to see the dynamic movements of voices and what a voice hearer could learn to do to change it can be a really helpful process. I need to develop assertiveness, but the nature of that assertiveness is specific to me and what another voice hearer may discover during the exercise will be very specific and personal to them.

I want to speak directly to voice hearers who struggle with being assertive in situations that would make a real difference to relationships with voices and in the world.

Above all, the voice mapping exercise may help break through a common, seemingly intransigent belief: "This is how it is"; "Voices are in charge, and I can do nothing about it". This can also reflect a life position, that others are in charge, or you need to give them a privileged position in your life and you don't have the power to do anything about that but accept this life-limiting position. Starting to chip away at this belief by taking an assertive position within a relational dynamic can help change the intrapsychic landscape with voices and may create a possibility that you can dare to take an increasingly assertive step in interpersonal relationships with others. This doesn't happen quickly but changing to a more assertive position with one voice may help to support an assertive position with someone in the world, and vice versa. It's a higgledy piggledy pathway but slowly, change, growth, and harmony can be established when it is reached for.

(Continued)

Table 7.1 (Continued)

Aligned with the Tripartite Relationship Theory, increasing your own assertiveness is synonymous with self-agency, which enables you good opportunities to influence the bullying aspects of your voices. Voices have many facets, and when you can look and get underneath the bullying energy, you may find these other qualities that can be directly helpful. Mapping your voices and exploring their movements and your impact on them, their impact on you, and the impact of the world on all of you can be a powerful way of discovering the specific answers you need to your particular situation and the distress related to it. Voices can be tremendous teachers and sign posters. Their demands that you assert yourself in the world can feel oppressive but can eventually do the paradoxical opposite and be liberating. Voice mapping isn't a magic wand to "fix" something but can be a powerful way to illuminate what a voice hearer struggles with and can pinpoint where to focus energy and intention to change something and create another step towards harmony with voices and harmony with self.

taking part in the activity and of the contribution this makes towards understanding and making changes to voice hearing experiences.

Concluding comments

The life map and voice mapping scenario we have discussed in this chapter illustrates an active and hostile relational context constructed by RL and in which power is threaded through interactions between RL and her voices and amongst her voices. Events taking place in RL's interpersonal context influenced both her intra- and inter-personal relationships. She had the opportunity to conclude that her struggle to assert herself interpersonally mirrored her struggle to assert herself with her voices, specifically Bill. Through engaging with her voices and trying a creative way of moving voices through the mapping activity, she demonstrated that she could change her voice hearing experience. We believe this empowering opportunity is possible for all people distressed by voice hearing. Through taking action, voice hearers can empower themselves to bring about positive change, even when experiencing difficult and distressing voice hearing experiences.

Chapter 8

Communicating with voices

Talking with voices and mark-making

We have so far discussed how we can gain a greater appreciation of voice hearing experiences through profiling and mapping voices in relation to a person hearing voices. We also illustrated how this can potentially help empower individuals to explore steps they might take to reclaim power from their voices to achieve greater harmony in their relating with their voices. In this chapter, we turn our attention to two methods we routinely utilise to communicate with voices: talking with voices (TwV) and mark-making. Through communicating with voices, we can further our understanding of them, including how and where they are experienced in relation to the voice hearer. As we have previously stated, we encourage a flexible and integrated approach to voice profiling (Chapter 6), voice mapping (Chapter 7), and communicating with voices, wherein each compliments and informs the other. We begin first with the TwV approach and then we discuss mark-making.

Talking with voices

Introduced in Chapter 2 and influenced by the Voice Dialogue method of Stone and Stone (1989) and rooted in the Hearing Voices Movement, TwV is a communication method that aims to facilitate ways of relating between an individual and their voices. In this chapter, we describe the practical steps we take during our workshops and then share our thoughts and experiences of engaging in this approach. It is important to note that individuals' voices are present even if others (i.e., practitioners and family members) haven't been aware of them, and the voices will observe, listen, and respond to the presence of others. Extending this, it is also important to note that other people contribute to an individual's voice hearing experience, for good or bad, but perhaps are not aware of it. Acknowledging this is at the heart of the Tripartite Relationship Theory. Being able to recognise this enables greater awareness and more explicit recognition of how one can make efforts to ensure they contribute to a positive experience.

Why talk with voices?

There are several reasons why it can be beneficial for a person to take part in this approach. For example, benefits can be experienced through getting to know each

DOI: 10.4324/9781032619910-11

voice, listening, and attempting to understand the meaning of their statements, their tone, to build trust with a hope that they can start to relate with the voice hearer with increasing respect and collaboration. Perhaps most importantly, it can aid the development of greater harmony and a more peaceful relationship between an individual and their voices. Aligned with a broader relational approach, the thesis of this book is that voice hearing can become less distressing and more harmonious through building more helpful ways of relating between an individual and their voices. An important contribution to relating is the building of a helpful relationship. This concerns the relationship between the voices and the voice hearer and amongst the different voices. To enable this, it is important to find a way of communicating, and the TwV approach provides one method of doing this.

Through TwV, more information can be learned regarding the reason for their existence and any meaning a voice hearer might associate with this, the voices' intentions, and their role in the voice hearer's life. The information acquired from these conversations can provide useful information that can be added to the voice profile and inform the life and voice mapping.

Building a relationship with voices and gaining greater appreciation of their perspective can enable the potential for individuals to reflect on their understanding of their voices. A common trait for us all is to form a conclusion about a range of things (i.e., people and events) based on relatively limited information. We are hard-wired to take cognitive shortcuts when trying to make sense of something and make a decision. Most, if not all, of you reading this book will have countless times experienced situations in which you jumped to a conclusion about something without fully taking into account all the relevant information. For example, you might have formed an opinion about a person or a specific type of food or clothing that you liked or disliked only to discover at a later date that you changed your mind. Perhaps you took an immediate dislike to a colleague at work based on how they dressed or how they spoke or even perhaps due to something you couldn't quite articulate, only to realise later after getting to know the person that they aren't quite as dislikeable as you first thought, or even that you actually liked them. Maybe you reflected that the initial opinion you made about your colleague was largely informed by your previous experience of knowing someone you thought was similar and the memory from that other similar person clouded the opinion you had formed regarding your colleague. Or perhaps you learned more about your colleague to help you better understand why you had formed your opinion, and you can now explain this more clearly to yourself. Having conversations with voices, and permitting others to have conversations with voices, can provide valuable opportunities to check whether initial opinions remain true even after learning more about a voice.

Extending the above, whilst it is perfectly understandable that voice hearers might repel their voices, for example, they might feel sickened at the presence of their voices or upon hearing what they say, it is also important to remember that this response is based on the meaning associated with voices and the subsequent interpretations made by the voice hearer concerning them. This is informed by the evidence the voice hearer has gathered about their voices. As such, there is potential for more information to be gathered and to be used by the voice hearer to form a different opinion about voices that potentially challenge initial impressions formed about them. Changing the relationship between the individual and their voices also offers the potential for this to become one that is perceived to be more peaceful and less distressing. This, in turn, offers an opportunity for a voice and a voice hearer to become more helpful to one another. This can be an important contribution to the overall voice hearing experience in which some voices might be experienced as a "personal bully" (Tripartite Relationship Theory) and those voices that are perceived as being or becoming more helpful can become an ally to the voice hearer to help them to manage their voice-related distress.

Finally, it offers an opportunity for greater integration between individuals and their voices. In doing so, voice hearers have an opportunity to reflect on the connection between their inter-personal and intra-personal contexts and explore ways to take greater control of these. This can positively impact the "level of agency" and "interpersonal dynamic" (Tripartite Relationship Theory). Included in this, voice hearers can explore opportunities through the TwV approach to learn not only more details concerning the intentions of voices but also how to communicate in a way that contributes to greater harmony intra-personally and mirror this in their inter-personal relationships. For example, if a voice hearer experiences situations in which they struggle to assert themselves with another person and then, additionally, experience hostility from their voices, they might conclude that they can reduce this hostility with their voices by developing more assertive ways of communicating with this other person (linked with the voice mapping exercise in Chapter 7). RL offers her reflection on her experience below (Box 8.1) of engaging in this approach.

Box 8.1   RL's experience of the TwV approach

I had been hearing voices for about two years and, on reflection, I wanted to move from a startle phase to a more organised and productive way of living with voices.

I signed up to a workshop led by Ron Coleman, Dirk Corstens, and Eleanor Longdon. They talked about how real voices are and what they may represent. This quest of discovery included talking with a voice. Kate was a mental health nurse who had joined the workshop to learn more about voice hearing. When it came to the TwV practice, I was paired with her. She was respectful and kind. I was anxious and I'm sure she was too. Kate introduced herself to my voices and asked if any of my voices wanted to have a conversation with her. We didn't know each other but I intuited the generosity she offered was neither a voyeuristic interest nor a trick to get this unusual phenomenon to emerge. These had been some of my fears about attending the course. This may be many people's concerns when they are thinking about talking with a voice. Voices will probably also have this same concern. They may fear being tricked, coerced, or disrespected. Distressed voices also tend to be suspicious because they don't want to experience any further distress. Equally, they may also be desperate to talk for themselves, directly to someone other than their voice hearer.

An additional fear was that I wouldn't be able to regain control of the conversation. If I let a voice speak, would they take over and would I be forever silenced and take the place of a voice, calling out in the mind of another but not audible to the rest of the world? It was this thought, the first empathic consideration that I had had towards my voices, that helped me make the decision to try and let them talk with another person other than me.

In introducing herself to my voices without any idea of who may reply, Kate made herself vulnerable. I appreciated her courage, and this allowed some of my anxiety to dissipate and think about who may want to speak. At the time, the first voice I started to hear, who I variously called "number one", "my first voice", or "my dominant voice" was very present with what felt like an urgent energy. He didn't say he wanted to speak with Kate because, at that time, none of my voices spoke in a direct way. I experienced them as unpredictable, speaking randomly, usually acutely offensively. A bit feral if I'm honest and I apologise to all my voices as I write this but that was how I experienced them. They were not my friends. I had a partial hope that talking with them may dissolve their energy and they would disappear. I also suspected that they were here to stay or at least would always have a more dynamic presence than something that could be wished away by releasing some negative energy through a few conversations with them. I also heard something in the workshop that made tremendous sense to me and that I took seriously. Voices were vocalising something authentic as a consequence of something that had happened to me. I made the connection that these things had happened to them too. I felt a bit more empathy for them.

This new insight was important but wasn't sufficient to quell my fear of them in a conversation with another. How could I allow this very bombastic, controlling, and critical, sweary voice to speak to this kind woman called Kate? I spoke my concern about his language and attitude. She seemed unphased. What was I to do? Stay safe and say there was no one who wanted to speak or take a risk. I couldn't make it any worse. I stood back and slightly to the left in my own space because that was where I sensed my first voice was. I nodded to Kate.

Kate introduced herself and asked if anyone wanted to speak with her. I don't recall the content of the conversation, but I know my first voice introduced himself as Grande. He had a job to do and that I (RL) was a "fuckwit". I recall Kate thanking Grande for speaking with her and that she hoped his experience of speaking with her was ok. For fear of repeating myself, her respect for Grande, including her tolerance of the profane term of reference that he used, and the non-coercive quality of her questions and invitations were pivotal in creating a space for Grande to emerge in an authentic, if defensive and strongly assertive way, but not with the uncontrolled aggression that I feared he might or that I experienced alone in my personal space with him. It could be argued that the term "fuckwit" was aggressive, and it is, but in relation to the need to make contact with a voice where they are, I feel it's necessary for me to tolerate the profanity, if the person speaking with my voice can tolerate it. The raw language dissipates in time and can be negotiated if it doesn't.

This was the start of a way of living with my voices, constantly moving to a way of sharing the living space, negotiating time for them and time for me, consulting them, and now listening to their advice and wisdom. I now have regular TwV conversations. I imagine people who hear a voice that they may want to speak with have a fear of their voice's power. I used to have a lot of fear about the power of the voice to negatively affect me, and as importantly for me, I feared them negatively impacting the person they would speak to. I don't like to hear my voices speaking with coarse or disrespectful words when speaking with another and so I negotiate with them to not use these words. This helps me feel more comfortable and confident and also helps build the ever-needful assertiveness and self-agency skills. I emphasise this as I think this is probably a common concern. I also know a common fear is being overpowered by the voice and by allowing them to speak, then a voice hearer is giving even more ground to them. I understand this fear, and whilst I have disproved this to myself with some of my voices, there is still a voice that I am reluctant to enter into a TwV conversation and the fear of giving him more power than I think he has already is part of it. However, I am moving towards engaging more fully with this voice and I discuss this with Grande and other voices. Currently, Grande is very unhappy about this. His wisdom is important to me, as is his own anxiety so I defer but holding that this may be something we both may agree to do in the future. I also believe that giving voices a space to speak diffuses some of the aggression that I can confuse with a desire for power and control. Their aggression is almost exclusively related to raw pain from previous life experiences, and when I remind myself of this, it helps me see beyond their words and helps me see their energy in the complexity that it represents. Talking through these concerns with people you trust is important. The most helpful environment for these discussions is in a well-run Hearing Voices Group (HVG) or with a practitioner who has some understanding of the hearing voices experience.

In terms of what the experience feels like, it feels odd! Voices generally feel like "other", even if the voice hearer believes, as I do, that voices are part of the whole self. The first occasions of a voice speaking to someone else can also be anxiety provoking because of the range of personal doubts and concerns they may have. The value of tolerating this oddness and discomfort is in getting to know and understand each individual voice and that over time the conversations become more and more sophisticated. For example, with my relationship with Grande, the conversations he can have with another have allowed him to be a separate self and able to show me more directly what his concerns and purposes are and what he thinks of me and what he would like me to hear and take seriously. These conversations are different from the kind that we have just he and I. They have a more boundaried and purposeful quality. We can now have more purposeful conversations alone, but I do not think that would have been as easy to establish without the involvement of others for him to talk to and for me to hear. Getting to know Grande in a more rounded way through his communication with others has enabled me to see who he is as a relational self. This has allowed me to enrich my experience and understanding of him and consequently has allowed him to communicate more directly, in the context of a growing, respectful relationship. We can relate and negotiate and live together rather than despite each other. We co-create harmony on a daily basis.

How to talk with voices

We have found that voice hearers, understandably, can feel anxious about the idea of either themselves or another person talking with their voice(s). Many might talk *at* their voices and perhaps react frustratingly to them but feel much less confident at the prospect of engaging in a more formal conversation *with* their voices. During our workshops, we have also found that voice hearers new to the TwV approach are interested to observe the process, but understandably hesitant to try this for themselves, especially in a workshop environment. Some people might have either observed or taken part in this during an HVG, which we consider to be a supportive environment for those who might be interested in exploring this further. Arguably, HVGs provide more opportunity than workshops to provide more time to develop trust and familiarity with other group members, to feel supported and have an opportunity to come back regularly to explore further and to learn from undertaking the approach at the voice hearer's pace, level of confidence, and trust. We offer the following steps with this in mind and acknowledge the potential difficulty for anyone interested in pursuing this, and we offer this only as a guidance based on what we have learned from others and through our own application.

Identifying a voice for a conversation

It is important to first ask the person hearing voices whether any are present and interested in having a conversation with another person. This might be simply a matter of asking the individual whether any of their voices are around, perhaps listening in or observing things taking place, and whether they are interested in taking part in a conversation with the other person (i.e., practitioner, family member, and friend). If more than one voice is interested or would like to take part, then we suggest a decision ought to be made regarding which voice to talk with first. It might become clearer shortly why we only converse with one voice at a time but, for this part, we suggest you work with one at a time.

Selecting which voice to talk with is a personal choice and the decision should be made by the voice hearer. It is likely that some voices will feel less threatening, and therefore less anxiety-provoking, than others; or that some voices might intuitively feel like a more natural choice than others. Some might prefer to first talk with voices that are considered to act as a protector of some sort for the voice hearer, which intuitively makes sense given the protection they might be perceived as providing for the voice hearer. If this is familiar to the individual, then they may also like to utilise this approach for other voices too, perhaps voices that are less protective and more hostile but important to engage with to help bring harmony more systemically amongst all the voices. There might not necessarily be a "right" or "wrong" choice, but we suggest you consider making your decision with an attitude of wanting to learn more about voice hearing experiences and an aim to reduce tension and related distress in the voice hearer-voice relationship.

Clarifying the purpose of a conversation with voices

After a decision has been made regarding which voice to talk with, we suggest the voice hearer and the other person involved in the TwV approach agree on the purpose of the conversation. For example, if this is the first time using this approach, then it would be helpful for the person talking to the voice to focus on introducing themselves to the voice e.g., enquire about the voice, ask for their name if there hasn't been one already provided, or ask the voice about their purpose. There are helpful guides and prompts available online, for example, May and Svanholmer (2019) have produced a self-help guide to TwV that readers can refer to for further suggestions when using this approach. We provide an example of a conversation in Box 8.2. Typically, we discuss the purpose before we use this approach so that we can be clearer whether there is a particular new issue RL would like to explore, or if there is something to flag up and avoid, or whether there is something from previous conversations that would be helpful to explore further.

Starting the conversation

An observation from our workshops and the support we provide to practitioners in clinical practice is that it can be difficult to know how to start a conversation with a voice. It can be difficult from the voice hearer's perspective, as we previously touched upon, and also for the other person, who typically might struggle to know how they are going to meet a voice and what they will then say to the voice. They may wonder whether they should summon a voice or just wait for something to happen. It may differ for individuals but, in our experience, the voice hearer knows if a voice wants to speak, and they make a conscious decision to let the voice speak through the voice hearer. When RA talks with one of RL's voices, he typically asks if RL and the selected voice are ready and then asks if RL can allow the voice, for example, Grande, to come into the foreground of her relational space so that he can begin a conversation with RA. Grande will then speak through RL and a conversation then begins. When the conversation comes to an end, RA then thanks Grande for the conversation and asks if RL can come back into the foreground.

Noticeable physical changes during the TwV approach

For people who have never observed someone talk with another person's voices before, it can appear a little unusual to observe, if only at first. Although this might not always be the case, there are typically two striking changes to the voice hearer's presentation. First, their physical energy can be noticeably different from their usual state. For example, they might ordinarily present as calm, they might have been sitting slouched, and they might have a quiet demeanour; this can change dramatically, depending on the energy of the specific voice. For example, with the voice now present in the conversation, the voice hearer might stand (where before they sat), they may present as much more energetic with the chest more open and the shoulders back, and they may go to a different place in the room. Second, the sound of the voice (i.e., Grande) can change and be noticeably different for others to hear. For example, the voice might sound louder, use different language, or have a different intonation, pitch, or pace. When the conversation with the voice ends, it is also striking to observe further changes associated with the return of the voice hearer, e.g., further changes to their physical energy, changes to the sound of their own voice, and possibly even changes to where they position themselves in the room.

Summary and discussion after a conversation with voices

Upon completion, the person involved in talking with a voice requests the voice hearer to return. For those who haven't yet observed this approach, this is not to say the voice hearer physically disappears and then reappears. Their voices speak through them. They might move to a different position and present with different energy and sound different, but they remain in the room. Rather, we essentially mean for the voice hearer to take back control and speak with their own voice. Some people might dissociate during this process, where they can feel mentally detached from their physical self and from the situation. Indeed, some people might have little or no recollection of the conversation that had taken place between one of their voices and another (third) person. In these situations, it is important for the third person to summarise the conversation for the voice hearer.

When RL and RA undertake this approach, RA will typically check with RL whether she heard the conversation between RA and her selected voice and whether a summary of it is required. During our early days of utilising the TwV approach, RL was not able to recall all discussions between RA and her voices and so it was common practice for RA to provide a summary of the discussion. For the past several years, however, this has changed to the point where RL is able to recall TwV conversations, making it unnecessary to provide a summary.

After it has been established whether a summary is needed (and, if so, this is then provided), we advocate taking a few moments for the voice hearer and third person to reflect on the TwV conversation. This helps provide space for further thinking about things voices say, to explore possible meanings associated with the content of the conversation and possible actions to consider in relation to this, and to consider possible helpful topics to discuss or questions to ask in future conversations with voices.

Box 8.2   RL's reflections of involving a third person in conversations with voices

Having a third person for your voices to talk with changes the experience of hearing them, whilst they are speaking to another person. Introducing a third person into a conversation with a voice can change the direction of conversations similar to the way a third person can when two people become stuck in their relationship. The extent to how much this might change experiences of voice hearing depends on the voice hearer, the voice, and where they are in their patterns of relating with the other person.

Imagine a situation where two people (or a family) have no choice but to live in the same house but do not get on with or understand each other and, despite one or all trying to resolve this, they struggle to find a peaceful way to negotiate their differences. They might even perceive their situation to be so different that they seem to speak a different language to one another. If neither can understand the other's heated statements and replies, the house would become dominated by friction, frustration, anxiety, anger, and avoidance. A third person entering into this dynamic and being equally respectful of all those who live in the household can bring new energy, a fresh perspective, and loosen up some of the friction between them. Their entry into the conversation can often enable the family to talk to each other differently. Relating this to voice hearing, from personal experience, introducing a third person into conversations with voices can similarly be helpful. Here are some examples of the valuable things that voice hearers can experience from their voice talking with a third person:

- A third person can endorse the reality of a voice, which, as we have previously discussed in relation to Romme and Escher's seminal work, can be important and helpful to the voice hearer and significantly to the voice.
- Similar to how voice profiling and voice mapping offer space for reflection on voices by recording details about them, a third person engaging in a conversation with a voice enables distance from the voice. This may be experienced as unusual as the conversation happens from within you and you may typically hear your voice in the room or at a distance rather than inside your head. The distance we mean is the relational distance. Talking with someone is different to hearing a conversation between two people. If you can be present

during the conversation, it is more possible to think about the conversation, what was said, and what the voice might have meant. If you are not fully present, the summary your third person offers about the conversation can importantly help you to reflect and add to the information and understanding you have of that voice.

- Voice hearers can be a witness to the conversation rather than the person being spoken to or talked at. You may hear yourself being spoken about and this is different from being spoken to.

- Empathy and understanding of the voice hearing experience can increase both from the perspective of the person who is talking with the voice and the voice hearer towards the voice and themselves. Another person has a direct experience of your invisible voice, which can increase their empathy and understanding of not only your experience but also voices' experiences of living with you/a voice hearer. When viewing this from the perspective of the Tripartite Relationship Theory, this exchange and effort to understand can improve the interpersonal relating and offers the voice hearer and voices opportunities to make their own sense of each other a little more.

- The conversation with a third person changes the experience of hearing your voice, which in and of itself can help a voice hearer develop a different perspective. This can help them develop a deeper understanding of their voice as a relational entity rather than as a disembodied voice.

- Introducing a third person into a conversation always changes the relational dynamic. A conversation between two people is very different to a conversation that includes a third person that is formally invited. When the third person is truly respectful of both voice and voice hearer, they can both experience having someone in their corner and witness the other being respected too. RL will return to this shortly to discuss how vital this point is in lowering friction and bringing a quotient of harmony to the relationship between voice and voice hearer.

Mark-making as a way to communicate with voices

Having discussed how to communicate with voices through a verbal conversation, we turn our attention to another method we believe is both alternative and complimentary to the TwV approach. This concerns an approach that emerged from a pathway of discovery for one of us (RL) that led to engaging with a voice, not through the use of words but exchanging marks on paper. This is a different way of having a conversation with a voice and has the potential to allow expression of the unspeakable as well as aspects of the relationship a voice hearer has with a particular voice. The aim, as with TwV, is to understand the specific nature and relationship with a voice, to get to know the voice more deeply, to improve harmony between voice hearer and voice.

Mark-making with a voice was a personal discovery that RL made whilst muddling through a piece of artwork required for submission to a Master of Arts (MA) Art Course. There are many forms of art therapy that use mark-making to explore aspects of self and relationships. Some voice hearers use art to explore their feelings, draw their voices, and explore their energy and conflicts. Although the act of mark-making is not an original technique, and some people might have found this or similar ways of communicating with their voices for themselves, to our knowledge no previous research evidence has utilised this specifically as a method to communicate with voices. RL, therefore, does not at all declare it as her invention with a voice, but it is a personal discovery.

This approach emerged from making deliberate pieces of art. However, mark-making with a voice is not about making a piece of elaborate art but can be about a number of intentions: playing to see what emerges; exploring a stuck point with a voice that doesn't seem resolvable by talking; sharing an experience and so resonating with each other in a way that can't be articulated. The end result is a recording of the non-verbal conversation. No artistic skill or expensive equipment is necessary; a piece of paper or flipchart, a pencil and perhaps some coloured pens or crayons and perhaps most effective, chalk pastels are all that are needed. The shapes and symbols, words or lines, whatever the voice hearer and the voice spontaneously make to communicate with each other is the intention. A pleasing or meaningful piece of abstract or figurative art may emerge, of course, if that is how the voice hearer or voice defines it; it can be as simple or as complex as they like. It is for the voice hearer and voice to decide and experiment with.

What follows is a personal account of RL's journey into what became a creative practice and how some of her voices responded to the decision to start learning how to make art. As with any significant change voice hearers make in their life, voices respond in their own way. This is a description of how RL's voices responded and how she discovered a way of communicating with her voices in a new way. The sharing of this personal journey is to encourage others to own their own path to explore aspects of their own life in a creative way and discover their own specific freedoms and solutions and find ways to communicate more effectively with their voices in ways that are unique to themselves and their voices. If a voice hearer likes writing, poetry, dancing, playing sports, or making music, anything that is an expression of the true self, then there are potential ways of collaborating with voices through these mediums to gain a greater satisfaction in life with voices. If you like to write, then maybe a voice may write something new, if you like to dance, maybe a voice may want to dance. Exploring and playing can bring a vitality and a mutual connection that may help breach the cavernous gaps between voice hearer and voice.

Making art is a primal way to express a moment in time, to communicate something, and to leave a mark in the world as a symbol of the experience. We are modulated by our experiences and mark-making provides a connection with learning who voices are and how they emerge. Our life events write themselves into our way of being and sculpt who we are and so exploring relationships with voices through making marks rings with a possibility of discovering something together that speaks of the past and present and enables the construction of something new. RL has faith that if her voices are a creative solution to old and ongoing challenges, then the creativity of the present may help her use new ways to evolve with her voices towards a more stable and synchronous path.

The start of the journey

Before embarking on her mark-making journey, RL had utilised the TwV approach with two of her voices over several years, learning who and why they were. The increased stability she had slowly built during this period enabled her to consider applying for an MA Art course, which she began, and which subsequently provided opportunities to explore many forms of creative practice: drawing; painting; making images; and forms with all sorts of materials such as wool, handmade paper, clay, and drinking straws! It turned out to be a divine playground. The course tutors were safe, encouraging, and generous in sharing their ideas with all the different students with their various interests and strengths. The combination of a safe place with enough safe people and the excitement of exploring something so meaningful to RL bolstered her confidence and ability to connect her emerging artistic skills to old crafting skills to make something new. It was exciting and challenging every day. She knew this was the start of a new and important phase of her life. One she had very deliberately chosen and wanted, which is significant in relation to what happened with one of her voices.

Upon starting the course, one of her voices, D, who usually had less to say than her primary voices, began to move closer and talked voluminously. Not aggressively, his energy was calm but keenly interested, and not directly about the course or RL's hesitant steps in exploring these new places and materials, but about seemingly random things that he hadn't talked about before. In the past, exchanges between RL and D were generally fractious, conflicted, and marked by mutual frustration. RL hadn't been able to work out what he wanted from her and always felt D experienced her as misunderstanding him. She experienced him as disgusted and impatient, and he didn't respond to enquiries about his role in the way that Grande or George did. RL had talked to D many times on her own but had never involved a third person utilising the TwV approach. Possibly, this may have elicited a more fruitful conversation, as with Grande and George. D shifted his way of talking to RL to the point that she wondered if a new voice had emerged; he had a characteristic voice with a recognisable tension and drive in his tone. Now he was talking about the weather and the things he saw, and his style of talking changing to more of a commentary. He didn't seem to be seeking RL's attention for all the things that had previously frustrated him. Feeling immersed in the art course, RL didn't pay too much attention to him at the time but did note the shift in his way of coming at her and the world. She registered how much easier he was to have around and planned to make some time for him. She was a few weeks into the course before she realised he had stopped talking about a week previously and he hasn't spoken since. Why? Why had there been this change and why did he no longer talk? Why, when we just seemed to be walking along together without the friction, did he stop talking? In current reflection, the obvious conclusion is that he had done his job, perhaps. RL's acting upon an impulse that was congruent with herself and her nature perhaps was sufficient for D to rest and cease to clamour for the attention to this particular aspect of RL's need to use self-agency. Voices always have the potential to return, but for now, there is less volatility in the space around her, and her assertive action has brought some degrees of harmony and perhaps a resolution.

Discovery of collaborative mark-making with Grande

After RL had decided to learn and apply herself to her artwork and D had become silent, another process began to evolve with Grande, a voice with whom she has the most communication and the most sophisticated relationship. Although her relationship with Grande had already begun to improve markedly through the TwV approach, he could still become agitated and RL would regularly make time to listen to and attempt to understand what Grande was trying to tell her. His concerns were usually about the emotional content of the day or his ongoing conflicts with RL and other voices. After about 18 months into the art course, she had discovered a style of print making that she identified as her medium and was starting to pursue this more seriously She was nearing a submission date and concerned to do her best. Grande was particularly agitated one morning as RL was designing a print. He wasn't responding to requests to contain his concerns to discuss later in the day and her frustration with him was increasing as she wanted her time and energy to be directed at her submission pieces. She spontaneously, and with some passive aggression, asked Grande if he wanted to draw a mark on the board she had been preparing to work on. She caught herself feeling exasperated and stopped. She knew that coming at her voices with dismissive frustration confounds the conversation and exacerbates their frustration. The retort to Grande, although flippant, bore an idea that maybe he would like to make a mark on the printing board. He may be amenable in the same way he was to talking with another person. She reminded herself that Grande more and more proved to be a protective energy and so she asked him again, from an authentic place of enquiry, whether he wanted to make a mark of his own. She didn't think too much about how it would work but just went with the idea and the invitation.

The following section (Box 8.3) describes a recollection of the conversation RL had with Grande during the first joint mark-making, partly verbal and partly through the exchange of marks on a printing board. You will note that parts of the conversation do not sound harmonious and include what can be regarded as abusive terms. It is useful to recall here the Tripartite Relationship Theory, in which the Personal Bully encapsulates features of many people's voices transactions and energy. Whilst rejecting the literal meanings of derogatory words and not attaching to them but rather tolerating them in order to understand the fuller intention of the communication, a more helpful way forward can be forged if there is a desire to genuinely understand a voice.

These oppressive-sounding transactions are included in the transcript below because they reflect the reality of many people who live with distressing and distressed voices. Some of the elements have been edited to protect the integrity of RL's relationship with Grande but include the significant transactions that are pertinent to demonstrating the process of working through some raw conflict. RL has found that tolerating the difficult language and energy is often a necessary step to develop mutual understanding, with a hope that the expression and acceptance of this energy start to be owned by both the voice hearer and the voice and aid the steps towards healing (Figure 8.1).

Box 8.3   RL's marking-making interaction with Grande and personal reflections (written in first person)

Day 1 of Mark-Making with Grande

RL: "Would you like to make a mark on the board, Grande?"
Grande: "No"

Grande said "No" very emphatically, but I felt a surge of energy in my hand and shoulder. I was holding a pencil and I experienced Grande make a very deliberate and energetic gestural line from right to left on the board. This surprised and excited me but made me quite nervous.

RL: "Are you cross with me?"

I asked this because I felt an angry energy in the making of the mark. I also replied specifically to the mark and drew two square shapes at the bottom of the board.

Grande: "Stop being a wimp"

Grande shouted loudly but also responded with some scribbly emphatic lines across the top of the board, again mostly left to right and back again.

RL: "What am I being a wimp about, Grande?"

Grande made no further verbal responses, but we continued a conversation on the board. We moved from pencil lines, which I later cut into on the board to make them more definite for printing, and we started using other materials such as paint, pva glue, and various bits of collage material.

Day 2 of Mark-Making with Grande

On the second day, I asked Grande again about the reference to being a wimp. As he made no verbal reply, I asked him if he wanted to reply with a mark. I suggested he could choose and make marks with glue, paint or pencil again. I picked up a tube of pva glue and felt his energy. The marks were scribbly, then splodgy and then more lines which became larger, slower and more flowing. I commented that I wanted to understand his frustration and that sometimes his cursing and insults could make me feel like I wanted to tear my hair out. I found a hairbrush and extracted some hair and stuck it on some of the lines of glue that he first made and then used some carborundum grit to spread over the other looping lines of glue. I generally used to feel guilty or anxious when I answered Grande back. My hair was now stuck on the board as a statement of my own frustration in relation to his frustration with me. A symbol of the aspect of our relationship that was still conflicted. I also wanted to acknowledge his frustration and talked to him about the lines of grit, that they would show up on the final print as very dark and I stated clearly that I wanted to acknowledge the seriousness of his frustration, that they left a mark on me too and I wanted to understand and learn from him. I then replied to his glue marks with my own. I put a gluey halo around the two square shapes at the bottom of the board and stated to him that I thought our relationship was important. He replied verbally:

Grande: "You've put us at the bottom and in the corner, you arse! You know nothing"

After some thought and temporary defeat, I replied.

RL: "I put them at the bottom because our relationship under-pins a lot of what is important in my life"
Grande: "Don't fucking appease me, you witch"

I thought some more and realised he was correct. I was trying to appease him. On reflection, I think it was an attempt to placate Grande as the risk of provoking and tolerating anger is still an issue I work with. It was also an attempt to relate and include both of us in the image, working and living in the same process and frame. Grande was not placated. Placating is an energy that does not come from a place in the self that is authentic but an aspect of being submissive, discounting one's own power. Over the years I have noticed that Grande can get adversarial when I communicate from this place either with him, other voices or in the world. When I find a way of staying in a balanced place where I can respect my own self agency, he speaks respectfully or not at all. I read this as him reinforcing only my authentic energy and very aggressively or firmly rebuking me when I communicate from a "one down" or submissive position. His energy and my energy are balanced when I am in a calm and assertive position. My anxiety that emerges when I adopt a "one down" place, triggers an aggressive "one up" energy from Grande. I reason that he is provoking me to strength by calling me "weak" etc. Over time I realise that one of the roles voices take up is to offer an opportunity to practice boundary setting from an Adult energy, and then dare to do the same in the world. I can practice standing up to voices and so to others in the world and vice versa.

I used to feel really intimidated by Grande when he was angry and seemingly unpredictable. I could have read his "don't appease me" statement as purely insulting or oppressive, but we had started a different kind of conversation and I wanted to do the same as I do when we just talk. To persist and try find a point of understanding, I reminded myself of my belief that Grande is essentially here to protect me and that often means protecting me from myself. Grande shows strong aggression when I do or say anything that disempowers myself. His fractious energy and statement indirectly invited me to respond in a more authentic way. I picked up the glue and splodged an abstract shape.

RL: "Your words are oppressive and sometimes I feel like you squash me into a corner with them".

I felt some anxiety at being so direct with him. I hadn't said it in anger or from a place of being a victim but from a place of being a bit cross but clear and factual. Assertive. I filled in the splodgy shape and covered it in carborundum grit (the grit soaks into the glue to make a dark line or shape once it has dried out). Grande didn't make a verbal reply to my spoken statement. I asked if he wanted to make another mark on the board. He remained silent. I took this as a positive thing in as much as he didn't need to justify himself but was quietly satisfied with the position I had taken with him and myself. More and more, I believe the words, whilst powerful, are not as important as the energy I use when relating to him and to the world. He is calmer and I am calmer when I can speak and live from a place of authentic expression. Responding to a voice's bullying energy with either aggression or submission locks me and my voice into a vicious escalating cycle. When I can respond assertively, I and my voices calm down.

Day 3 of Mark-Making with Grande

On the third day I tipped the carborundum grit from the board to see what our conversation looked like on paper. I was also interested, from an artist perspective, to see how the composition was shaping up. Each new phase of printing reveals an unexpected form when you are new to it as I was. I was surprised to uncover a shape at the lower left-hand side of the board that resembled a huge mouth. This was the splodgy reply to Grande's "don't appease me" statement. This again gave us an opportunity to discuss the marks and what they may accidentally or unconsciously represent. I had a long conversation with Grande as a result of this form of a mouth appearing on the board. The elements of the conversation included:

- The oppressive quality of Grande and other voices when they are verbally aggressive, and how this increases my anxiety and decreases my capacity to deal with the day and with other voices and visions.
- The form being like a pictorial representation of a voice. Seeing a voice represented in this form made me think about how a voice is equally, or more at the mercy of the voice hearer's speech, decisions and actions in the world – this made me consider carefully that a voice may be so emphatic because speaking is the only avenue of power and agency in the voice hearers world.
- How we can both feel consumed by each other's energy when I feel dysregulated.
- How we both feel like screaming at each other or at the world.
- How much Grande feels he has to shout at other voices when they become agitated.

Later in the day, and in a fool hardy way (Grande just tutted at me as I wrote "fool hardy"!!) I suggested he used the ferrous metal paint. It is a difficult material to handle. The potential for it being splashed around the table and ruining other work and tools was a distinct possibility on reflection, but maybe the trust allowed Grande to direct the paint onto the board, mostly! I felt his energy as the lines and loops of the paint found their place on the board. It was messy but energetic. They overlayed some of the original marks that he had made previously, and a random blob of the paint added an eye to the large mouth form and gave it some more identity.

I asked him what kind of energy expressed these new lines and he laughed. This is a rare event! Grande doesn't laugh much and so I interpret the squiggly lines and loops as an expression of joy. I enjoyed his joy. It is a rare kind of connection with a voice. I was glad Grande had enjoyed the process and I experienced a growing understanding and underlining of the things I was learning about Grande and our relating.

This print was later exhibited at an exhibition. It is to my shame that I felt unable to equally credit Grande with the work. I do this here and now.

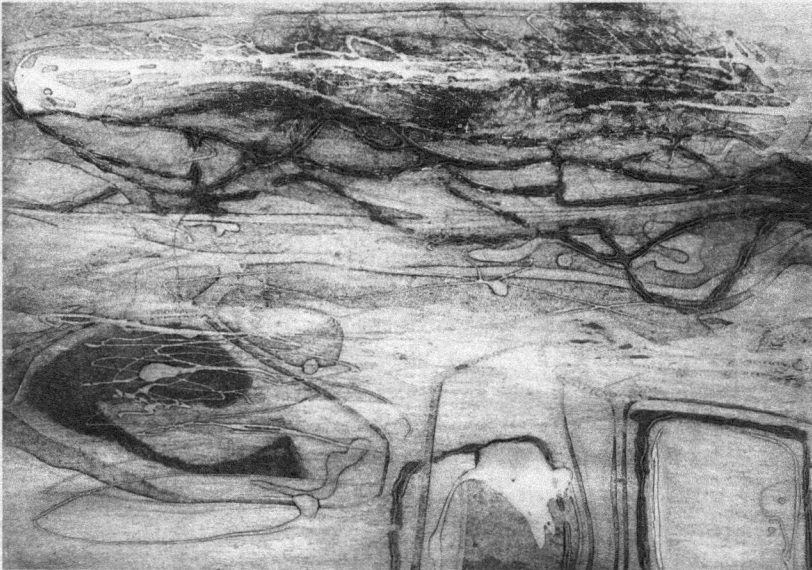

Figure 8.1 Chaos I, Ruth, and Grande (2018) Ink on Somerset paper.

The conversation on the print board had concluded with laughter and so I felt this was a finished piece. Once the board was sealed and I was able to print from it, choosing colours in collaboration with Grande, it rendered a piece of work from which we continued to have a verbal conversation, and several years on, we occasionally still do.

The final print is a tangible conversation. The elements can remind us both that we are in a creative relationship that allows both of us to speak about critical relational issues that not only impact us both but also affect how I relate to the people and issues in my world. The light and dark, the frustration, the "stuckness", pain and joy are all present and made visible. It is the record of a step in a journey. The mark-making gave us a collaborative team-building opportunity to get to know each other a little more and to represent a point of resolution. It slowed the conversation down and gave us both time to think about how to respond to each other and learn more about each other, as well as giving space to respond spontaneously and with authentic energy. I find it very difficult to be clear and state my reality verbally. I was able to speak through mark making and then that led to me being able to speak the words clearly. It was a prop to my assertive self. The resolution didn't fix something for good but boldly illuminated an important relational process and dynamic that I unconsciously repeat that causes Grande and I so much grief!

We were able to explore each other's feelings, thoughts, and beliefs. More profoundly, it enabled us to explore what it was like for each of us to be in relationship with the other. Starting to sound like couples counselling? It is, of sorts! It has a similar intention of helping to resolve difficulties in the relationship, to help each other hear, understand, and appreciate each other's position in the relationship with a hope of bringing a growing sense of equity and harmony. We used the mark making and the image as the mediator in a way.

I continue to have conversations through mark-making. I usually use this way of communicating when I find I am repeatedly getting stuck with a voice. It is flexible and has no technical rules. It can be purely mark exchanged with mark, talked about at the end with a voice, or not. It can be purely as a catharsis to express something and may not be possible for either the hearer or the voice to articulate. It can be a mark, followed by dialogue, as was my first experiment. Having "discovered" this, I was keen to explore it with RA. We now include this process in our training workshops.

Application of mark-making: guidance

For some, mark-making can be a less intimidating way of having a direct conversation with a voice but with the same intention of allowing space for the voice to express themselves and the voice hearer to reply through the mediator of the paper, chalk, pens, pencils, or crayons.

Many voice hearers already make art by, for example, drawing, painting, stitching textiles, or sculpting. This is a familiar activity for many voice hearers and may be done mindfully to reduce anxiety and so create a greater inner calm to cope with voices more effectively; indeed, voices may become less distressed when a hearer is more relaxed and focused. However, RL also recognises there are times when voices are at such a pitch that a focus on making art seems impossible.

Although mark-making might not always result in resolution for either voice hearers or their voices, expressing energy in this was can often be cathartic and subsequently lead to a calmer state of mind for the voice hearer to continue with their day with less intense interruptions from voices.

The beauty of mark-making on paper is that the conversation and themes held on the page can be something to come back to, make more marks, or have a discussion. It's a tangible object about which voice hearers can reflect when words are sometimes lost from recall. An important element of making a conversation visible is because much of what a voice hearer experiences can feel invisible, surreal. Sometimes it is hard to find the line between reality and unreality. Self-doubt about the reality of voices is something many voice hearers wrestle with. "Am I imagining this?", "are voices real?", "am I real?". Voice hearers are often met with comments from people who dismiss their voices. For example, RL recalls having to talk to a public servant who had asked her about her voice hearing, and he stated rolling his eyes "well I'm sure they're real to you", implying he thought they were not. This issue of reality is also significant for voice hearers who have experienced significant gas-lighting. The real elements of a conversation that remain recorded and that represent an authentic expression from a personal perspective and not reframed by another may also be an important way of recording a conversation. Mark-making with a voice does not solve this, but having a concrete image of a dialogue that a voice hearer can know is a real conversation with a real part of themselves may be important, just for that. Mark-making with voices is therefore a flexible way of communicating with voices. There are no strict rules to get right or wrong. It's about finding a personal way that works for each individual voice hearer and voice, in the moment.

Supporting a voice hearer to explore a voice or several voices through mark-making can be a helpful way to build trust between the supporter and the voice hearer and specifically their voices. Being alongside and interested in what voices have to "say" through their marks may provoke a number of emotional responses from a voice. This can include becoming more settled because they experience acknowledgement. It can also provoke suspicion or anxiety. These emotions are an important clue for the voice hearer to understand their voice in a more nuanced way, through exploring the interactions in this new creative situation. Giving space for these emotions to be expressed is really important as well as giving time at the end for the voice hearer to explore what their feelings and their voices expressed feelings were and what sense the voice hearer makes of them.

Helping to protect the time and space so that it is uninterrupted is useful to allow the voice hearer and voices to feel as safe as they are able to feel. Being present and quietly interested is a good stance to take during the process and to be encouraging to the voice hearer when the mark-making conversation is finished. Encouraging them to take their own time to think about what the marks on the page mean to them.

At this point, the key thing that we would stress more than anything to those supporting a voice hearer is to really hold onto the strong desire to interpret the marks and the images produced. It can feel fascinating and the urge to jump in and describe or define the marks can feel strong. Returning to the Tripartite Relationship Theory, this is an opportunity to support a voice hearer's agency to not only engage in the mark-making with a voice but also their opportunity to make their own sense of their mark-making conversation with their voice and to make a little more sense of the relationship with that voice or voices. The messages that can emerge through the marks can only be interpreted fully by the voice hearer and an early interpretation from another risks directing attention away from the importance of the messages on the page, diluting its potency, and frustrating the process of building a direct and meaningful moment of relating to the voice and the voice to the voice hearer. The roll of the practitioner or helper is to offer encouragement and support, not to take ownership of the process and thereby decommission the voice hearer's agency by declaring their own hunches about what the marks mean and how they were made. This can frustrate not only the communication but can also frustrate the voice. When a voice hearer has finished thinking and talking about the image, asking open questions about the elements of the image that strike you can be useful, however, and may add to the voice hearers understanding and endorses your interest in what the voice wishes to communicate. For example, you could ask about the colours that the voice has selected to make their marks with, and the colours the voice hearer chose to respond with. Asking about the relationship between the different marks or images can also be helpful if the voice hearer hasn't already made some connections with these elements. The rule of thumb is to enquire with open questions with the intention to increase a voice hearers search, rather than to find the message for the voice hearer. The treasure for the voice hearer is in discovering and realising the meanings for themselves.

Chapter summary

We have discussed two methods we typically utilise to communicate with voices: one involving a verbal conversation through introducing a third person into the voice hearer – voice relational dynamic and following the TwV approach and the other involving a mark-making activity between a voice hearer and voice. Both approaches can greatly enhance understanding of voices and the voice hearer – voice relationship – but are not without their challenges. Changing relationships can be very difficult for anyone. Furthermore, change often comes only through making sacrifices, i.e., giving something up to enable things to become different. We have provided examples throughout this and the previous chapters of situations in which one of us (RL) has been in that situation. For example, giving up a well-established, habitual way of relating in an interpersonal relationship with another person to help make changes to intra-personal relationships with voices; or letting go of attempts to control communications with a voice by permitting a third person to engage in conversations using the TwV approach; or sacrificing one's own time even when working towards a course deadline to explore ways of mark-making with a voice. Doing so, understandably, can evoke anxiety. In the next chapter, we discuss how to develop helping relationships to support making these changes.

Chapter 9

Nurturing helpful relationships

Relationships contribute in varying degrees to our lives: some people have many relationships in their lives, and some have very few. As we have discussed in the previous chapters regarding the Tripartite Relationship Theory, relationships concern people and also voices. Even if a person feels isolated and has minimal relationships with their voices, this is still a relationship of sorts. Although there can be some similarities, relationships between people are different from those with voices. An obvious difference is the ability to physically distance oneself from another person and end contact; however, one cannot so easily sever contact with their voices. They can't physically remove voices out of their lives in the same way they might with another person. They can, however, emotionally distance themselves from their voices, as we learnt from Bella's account in Chapter 3. You may remember, Bella termed a "minimal relating" way of being with her voices to account for her emotionally distant relationship with her voices. However, despite attempts such as Bella's to create emotional distance, voices are still there communicating to, or at, the voice hearer. So, the type of relationships we have in our lives matter greatly for our quality of life, including voice hearing experiences.

Indeed, the thesis of our book has concerned relationships at the interface between inter- and intra-personal relations and their influence on voice hearing experiences. At a primitive level, the development of effective relationships enabled humans to survive and evolve. Without the development of effective relationships and involvement of others in the lives of our predecessors, at the very least for support to hunt and gather food and for protection from predators, they (and consequently we) would not have survived. Life, as we know it today, is, of course, very different from earlier hunter-gatherer times, but the need to sustain ourselves (i.e., food, shelter, and protection) for our survival remains. We know from research evidence that exposure to threatening interpersonal relational situations, for example violence or bullying or neglect, increases the risk of developing voice hearing and a range of mental health difficulties. Conversely, relationships can be central to healing and good mental health where they are perceived as secure and comprise sufficient elements of trust. So, relationships are important to us all, although some of us may have good reason to give little if any recognition to them. But they remain central to voice hearing. For some people, perhaps with previous

DOI: 10.4324/9781032619910-12

experiences of difficult or even harmful relationships, life might have become a matter of getting through each day, surviving one day to the next. But is simply surviving enough? We may all have different ideas about what constitutes a happy life, and to what extent that involves others, but most voice hearers at the very least want to be at peace with their voices, to have harmonious relationships with their voices. In this penultimate chapter, we consolidate our ideas discussed throughout this book regarding how people who hear distressing voices can improve relationships that impact their voice hearing experiences.

In a clinical context, the onus of responsibility for developing positive relationships with patients is placed predominantly on practitioners. Their ability to develop helping 'therapeutic' relationships with patients is recognised in both research and professional-body literature as the cornerstone of effective care (Wood & Alsawy, 2016; Peplau, 1992, 1991). Their professional standards include developing trusting and respectful relationships with patients and promoting autonomy, empowerment, and shared decision-making during treatment (NMC, 2015; RCP, 2014; National Collaborating Centre for Mental Health, 2012). We notice this sense of professional responsibility transfer into our workshops. For example, an important question we are routinely asked during our workshops concerns whether the approaches we have shared throughout this book increase the risk for voice hearers. More specifically, practitioners can become worried about whether the application of these approaches increases the possibility that voice hearers might harm themselves or other people. From a clinical perspective, the approach to these concerns is couched as risk management, where the aim is to identify potential factors that contribute to the onset, exacerbation, containment and potential remedy of risk. Practitioners will therefore complete well-established assessments, part of a procedure they are expected by their employer to follow, to ensure that any risk has been identified and subsequently contained where needed. It is noteworthy, however, that there is mixed evidence regarding the use of formal risk assessment tools. A recent review (Saab et al., 2022) concluded they insufficiently predict risk and serve the needs of organisations rather than patients.

We do not wish to minimise concerns related to risk nor are we complacent towards the consequences of it. We are conscious of challenges associated with voice hearing specifically and emotional distress broadly. No doubt readers will also be too aware of examples reported in the media of tragic consequences when members of our communities have sadly become victims to the actions of individuals whose risk had not been effectively "managed".

Returning to our workshops, a specific concern expressed by practitioners specifically relates to whether the Talking with Voices (TwV) approach could lead to a voice hearer being harmed in some way. Understandably, practitioners (and families and other supporters) of course want to avoid making things worse for people who hear voices. They may feel anxious to avoid contributing in some way to voice hearers feeling more distressed, which may subsequently lead to them becoming a higher risk in terms of their own wellbeing and safety (and that of others). Arguably, risk can never be entirely eliminated; all involved can be left feeling anxious. Indeed, in some cases, healthcare services and practitioners have been accused of being risk-aversive. We believe it is important for practitioners and supporters to invest their energy in helping voice hearers to nurture helping relationships, both with self and others, as a way of building on their strengths to manage what might be referred to as risk. We explore this in more detail shortly.

You may recall in chapter two, we introduced the work of Romme, Escher and colleagues and the related Hearing Voices Movement. One of their key recommendations was for voice hearers to learn how to communicate effectively with their voices. To enable this, and align with our message throughout this book, voice hearers need to develop a relationship of some sort with their voices. For some, this will involve changing their relationship from one that causes distress to one that becomes harmonious. Throughout part three of this book, we have explained how this might be achieved through profiling, mapping, and communicating with voices. We have proposed through the Tripartite Relationship Theory that voice hearing experiences are influenced by not just practitioners, but also other people involved in, and supporters of, voice hearers.

Returning to the Tripartite Relationship Theory, we briefly recap some key points discussed in previous chapters regarding relationships and voice hearing. First, learning to engage with voices might be considered counterintuitive but can positively impact the voice hearing experience. People who are less distressed by their voices have established a way of being with their voices predicated on more helpful and harmonious relationships with their voices. Second, and to restate, voice hearing involves relationships both intra-personally with voices and interpersonally with other people. Both intra- and interpersonal relationships can impact on one another. Third, there is to some extent mirroring between intra- and interpersonal relationships for voice hearers. This essentially means where a voice hearer might struggle to assert themselves with other people, they might also struggle to assert themselves with their voices. Developing more agency to assert oneself with one's voices can support development of increased assertiveness with other people. This opens an important potential contribution from practitioners and supporters in terms of the role they can play to help improve voice hearer-voice relationships. Finally, as we have discussed throughout this book, relationships and power are intertwined. Relationships can be both disempowering and empowering in terms of voice hearing experiences, typically most explicitly observed through coercion, as we previously discussed in Chapter 2. For the remainder of this chapter, we return to the Tripartite Relationship Theory to frame our recommendations for nurturing helpful relationships.

Interpersonal dynamic

We have advocated throughout this book for increased harmony in relationships between voice hearers and their voices, with the aim of reducing relational hostility. However, as we have also discussed previously, voice hearing typically reflects difficult events (singular or a series) in the lives of the hearer, and which has involved a relational conflict of some sort with others. Given the potential for mirroring between interpersonal relations with other people and intra-personal relations with voices, which we illustrated during the voice mapping exercise in Chapter 7, it is important for practitioners and supporters to be self-aware regarding their own power dynamics and how this influences their own approach when relating with people who hear voices. We encourage voice hearers to develop assertive, respect-ful, and empathic relations with their voices and, to compliment this, we encourage voice hearers, practitioners, and supporters to communicate in a similar way with each other.

It is important that practitioners and supporters become confident in being with and listening to experiences of voice hearing. To aid this, we encourage practitioners and supporters to be reflexive regarding their relationships with people distressed by voice hearing. This includes being cognisant of the environment in which voice hearing is being experienced and to which they contribute and, therefore, how they might impact the voice hearing experience. It also means being aware of potential internal activity voice hearers can experience with their voices, especially during interpersonal social interactions. As such, we encourage practitioners and supporters to be self-aware regarding their verbal and non-verbal communications to help avoid potentially, and inadvertently, increasing distressing voice activity.

Practitioners and supporters can also help by looking for opportunities for non-threatening conversations with people about their voices. This should include always being respectful about and towards voices during conversations and talk-ing more openly about voices within the treatment environment (or at home, or wherever time is spent). For example, they could ask how the voices have been that morning, or if the voices (or even a specific voice by their name) are currently pre-sent (in the room) or if they have anything to say about a conversation that might have taken place or how they have been feeling. This does not have to be directed at voices or the individual hearing voices but could be an open question spoken out loud and simply asked out of curiosity. This helps to convey a message that the practitioner or supporter is accepting that voices are present and real, can be a way of validating the voices, and demonstrates they are interested to get to know the voices. It can also convey that they are not intending to be a threat to the voices.

Making sense

Rather than treat voice hearing as a symptom of a mental illness per se, instead we encourage approaches that help develop a personally meaningful understand-ing of voices and related difficulties. An understandable concern that many people have regarding voice hearing is the possibility of making things worse for a person hearing voices. Sometimes this extends to a real fear for the safety of the person hearing voices. What if they become so distressed they act on what their voices tell them to do? What if they hurt themselves or hurt somebody else? The sense a per-son makes regarding their voices is a large contributing factor to this concern. As we have discussed in earlier chapters, we encourage voice hearers to develop their own personal construction of their voice hearing experiences. To do so, they may benefit from engaging in opportunities outside of conventional mental health services, for example with other voice hearers in Hearing Voices Groups or alternative communities. To support this, it is important for voice hearers, practitioners, and supporters to review their own levels of knowledge and understanding about voice hearing and reflect on how they have come to know this and what other possible explanations there might be, and where they might be sought. Rather than impose expertise on a person distressed by voices, we encourage an open minded and curious approach to explore and understand individual experiences and explanations regarding voice hearing. In other words, avoid imposing pre-conceived beliefs and dominant narratives onto voice hearers but, instead, collectively explore potential roots to voice hearing experiences.

That said, some practitioners or supporters might have a question along the line of "what if a personally derived meaning regarding voices is associated with harming people", for example the voice is an omnipotent, omnipresent, and omniscient being that commands the voice hearer to harm self or others. This potential for harm is possibly central to most people's concerns regarding voice hearing and the responsibility placed on practitioners to manage the risks associated with this can cause conflict and tension when making decisions concerning how to respond to voice-related distress. We do not have the space here to do justice to this deeper, existential issue related to risk. Indeed, it is an issue about which we continue to develop our thinking as we learn more from our work. But we do want to offer our response to this concern.

We fundamentally believe in peaceful relationships. We have discussed throughout this book the underlying aim of the approaches we have presented is for voice hearers to develop harmonious relationships with their voices. We have also acknowledged that intra- and interpersonal relationships can be mirrored. Given this theoretical basis concerning relationships, we also stress the importance of harmony within interpersonal relationships. Indeed, this approach informed the voice mapping exercise discussed in Chapter 7. Therefore, we would challenge beliefs or personally derived meanings regarding voices that portray self or others as a target for harm. Where this cannot be controlled by individual voice hearers, we believe there is justification for practitioners to exert that control for the safety of the individual and/or other people. Typically, in some cases, this involves mental health legislation and medication.

Medication: helping or hindering?

Following the development of a meaningful understanding of voice hearing, there subsequently needs to be a logical link between this and the approaches taken to perhaps initially contain and then resolve any related distress. Putting aside issues related to the above discussion about risk, this ought to include the individual voice hearer's preferences regarding medication. In facilitating voice hearers to become involved in treatment decisions, it is important for opportunities to be created for dialogue between voice hearers, practitioners, and their supporters. These should also focus on how to resolve situations where disagreements might occur.

Extending the above recommendations related to making sense of voice hearing, practitioners and supporters need to reflect on what is meant by the term "treatment" and how medication contributes to this. This includes reflexivity concerning their own personal beliefs about voices and treatment, and how this might impact decision-making about the person distressed by voices. This returns us to the central role of power in respect of decisions made by practitioners/ supporters about another person distressed by voice hearing. Readers might recognise the intra-/interpersonal narrative here in terms of a voice hearer hearing commands from their voices but also hearing other people telling them what they are expected to do in response to their voice hearing and subsequent lifestyle. By permitting space for a voice hearer to own and make their own decisions about treatment, including taking into account potential consequences should decisions lead to further concerns, we believe individuals then have an opportunity to develop a sense of responsibility for their own treatment decisions and take ownership of the outcomes of these. Voice hearers can then aid their own recovery by exploring their own preferences about approaches to help improve their voice hearing experiences and how these might impact on their relationships with their voices.

Level of agency

Extending the point above, we move on to the notion of power. People who hear voices have typically survived situations in which they have experienced disempowerment, and from which their voices have emerged. Many who later struggle with voice hearing experiences encounter mental healthcare and receive treatment, typically medication as we have previously discussed. Many feel further disempowerment at this point of mental healthcare. In other words, earlier experiences of disempowerment and distress are compounded at a later point by further disempowerment from voice hearing and receipt of mental healthcare. As such, many voice hearers believe they have very little influence over their situation both intra-personally with their voices and interpersonally regarding their treatment. We believe a key element to improve voice hearing experiences is to improve the level of agency for people distressed by voices, as we have discussed in earlier chapters. We also believe it is important for people distressed by voice hearing to change difficult interpersonal relationships to help change their voice hearing experiences. This is not to say that other people in the life of a voice hearer make their voice hearing distressing. Rather, it is a situation in which they might struggle with an individual or people in general that is personal to them. Perhaps when they are in those situations, they are reminded of previous difficult times.

For example, you may hear voices and feel very distressed from hearing your voices, and at the same time also find yourself in difficult relationships with practitioners who are responding to your situation and distress. Or you may find yourself in a relationship with another person, perhaps a friend or partner, in which you struggle to assert yourself. This other person might be someone you love but, at the same time, you feel regularly compromised by their way of being with you. Perhaps, you find it difficult to say no to them, perhaps you feel you don't have enough space for yourself, and perhaps they sometimes behave in a way that upsets you. And perhaps you have felt unable to do anything to change this. We touched on this intra-inter-personal dynamic when we discussed voice mapping in Chapter 7. In our experience, in these kinds of situations, voices can become distressing for the hearer and, to expand on the "making sense" section above, one way of making sense of this is to consider whether the voices are signalling their disapproval and distress regarding the way in which you are feeling compromised in your interpersonal relationship. Of course, we are unable to "prove" this to be correct; meaning related to voices, after all, is constructed. If we do follow this line of thinking, however, it would suggest that addressing the feeling of compromise within the interpersonal relationship will positively impact voice hearing. To make such a change, though, can be difficult and we believe requires a reinforcement (or perhaps an introduction for some) of an interpersonal boundary between you and the other person. And this can be difficult. Most likely, you would have previously done this were it not so difficult.

To begin to address a difficult relationship, we strongly advise you to first be clear about what you want changing in the relationship. Pinpoint the specific behaviour that you find leads to you feeling disempowered. You may remember from the discussion on voice mapping that we commented that just because you want someone (or voices) to do something, or to stop doing something, doesn't mean they will. We may not be able to make others or voices do things, but we can learn how to express our needs and wants in a calm and assertive manner. Reclaiming and developing this part of oneself is an important element to building a personal level of agency.

To improve shared decision-making and voice hearing experiences more broadly, practitioners (and, where relevant, supporters) need to be aware of power imbalances within relationships. Power can be experienced as abusive, so it is important to be aware of the potential for relationships to be exposed to misuse of power. As such, it is important to be aware of potential contributions towards coercive practices, especially when administering medication or other approaches during interactions with voice hearers. Practitioners need to be reflexive regarding their role, and their perception of their role, within their team hierarchy and how this contributes to approaches taken to support people distressed by voice hearing. This includes developing an understanding of the concept of coercion, and how it is utilised in healthcare practice, and clearly differentiating this from the concept of choice.

Voice hearers would benefit from developing confidence to challenge coercion effectively and respectfully, both in terms of coercive practice administered by practitioners and their experiences of coercion with their voices. To support this, and to increase their levels of agency, we encourage voice hearers to make their needs, preferences and concerns clear to others and their voices, to take part in discussion and respectful debate rather than reluctant acceptance.

Chapter summary

Relationships can be complicated, complex, and challenging. For some, they can also be unpredictable and loaded with anticipatory fear of "what ifs", e.g., what if "they" try to hurt me, what if "they" don't like me or what I am doing, or even what if "they" leave me? In this respect, relationships can be accompanied by distressing emotions and worried thinking. It is unsurprising, then, in these circumstances that people who are already distressed by their voice hearing might find it difficult to be in a relationship and struggle to navigate their way round relationships. It is also important to hold onto the alternative view, however, that relationships can also be incredibly important. That is, they can be a source of support, they can enrich lives, they can bring happiness. As such, whether close or distant, relationships are meaningful and become a conduit of power. The thesis of this book concerns the role of relational harmony in the improvement in voice hearing experiences. To strive towards this goal, we believe in the value of focusing on strengths and building intra- and interpersonal helping relationships through a tripartite conceptualisation of voice hearing experiences.

Chapter 10

Concluding comments

As we approach the end of this book, in this final chapter, we want to reflect on what we hope you the readers will take from your reading to help you move forward and relate confidently with voice hearing. Before we began writing this book, we were clear that we wanted to embark on a journey through which we could further our own knowledge about voice hearing and one that would provide us with a platform to share some of our learning and experiences. It is important for us to be able to share knowledge and experience, the worth of which is always the chance that the information and life experiences we share can be useful to someone, that it offers new ways of looking at the dilemmas that voices and voice hearing present. We also wish to add our energy to the groundswell of change that is slowly impacting attitudes and perceptions of voice hearing both within services and the wider community. Being able to speak directly to voice hearers and supporters is a privilege and our hope is that voices are listening and considering what these chapters may offer them too.

We consider ourselves fortunate to have met many wonderful people over several years through our workshops, with whom we have collectively shared experiences and learnt from one another. We are thankful to everyone who attended. We are also thankful to all who shared their stories throughout the interviews and focus groups, which informed the development of the Tripartite Relationship Theory. We are also indebted to Rufus May, who kindly carved out time over several months to read through draft chapters and offer his reflections. Without the contributions of all those who have kindly contributed and shared their experiences, it would not have been possible to write this book. We hope it does justice to you all.

So, what do we hope you, the readers, will take from having read this book? Well, let's very briefly recap on the key take-home messages threaded throughout it. The first is to recall that voice hearing is not problematic *per se*. Many people hear voices but are not particularly troubled by them. Many people also hear a mix of voices, where some voices are troubling, but others are experienced positively. Readers will similarly have a range of different types of voices.

This leads us to the second take-home message, which influences how voices are experienced: voice hearing is about power. This concerns several areas but is largely rooted in relationships. This concerns either the way in which a person appraises

DOI: 10.4324/9781032619910-13

their voices (e.g., if the voice(s) are believed to be benevolent or malevolent) or how they relate to their voices (e.g., from a position of power or submissively). We expanded on this when we introduced the Tripartite Relationship Theory by introducing the role of intra- and inter-personal relating to account for the complex relational dynamic between a person and their voices and also a practitioner (or supporter). Power is recognised through a range of coercion, which is commonly reported in clinical contexts, and which is typically enacted through intra- and inter-personal relationships. For voice hearers, this concerns their relationships with their voices and with other people. Furthermore, power can be experienced and expressed through one's level of agency, both in terms of voice hearing experiences and concerning treatment-related decisions.

This leads us to the final take-home message, which concerns the way in which voices are experienced: voices can change. It might not seem plausible nor possible to those reading this who feel distressed by voice hearing. But it is an important message: voices can change; voice hearing experiences can improve. Voices emerge from personal experiences and so are rooted in voice hearers' history, the memories and interpretations of which subsequently shape the way the voices are constructed and recalled. Where many people might experience their voice(s) as a personal bully, through developing one's sense of agency, through improving relationships with others, through constructing meaningful explanations about voice hearing, and through determining if and how medication contributes to voice hearing experiences, this troubling experience can change to a much more positive one. Personal bullies can over time, and for many people do, become valued allies to the life of a voice hearer.

We have shared several approaches that can help facilitate this process of change, including voice profiling, life mapping, voice mapping, talking with voices, and mark-making. These are approaches that can become vehicles for improving relationships with voices but not an end point. The aim is not to get rid of voices. We have stressed throughout this book that our aim is to encourage harmony within intra- and inter-personal relations in order to develop peaceful relationships. In doing so, we consider intra-voice hearing experiences to be a barometer for inter-personal experiences. Through visiting and revisiting these exercises in an order that's right for each individual, reasons for voice-related distress can be illuminated and quelled.

Moving forward, we remind readers, and especially those distressed by voice hearing, to not only recognise that relationships are important, but that the quality of the relationship one has with oneself is the most important of all. We believe that accepting oneself without shame, valuing oneself despite a range of flaws we all have, helps improve intra-personal relationships with voices and inter-personal relationships with others.

What does improving your relationship with yourself look like? What does it mean? How possible is it? These are questions that are important for every single person. The answers are different for each person but are vital to ask. The difference for voice hearers is that the internal conflicts between different parts of ourselves are vocalised and enacted in a profoundly combative way. As voice hearers have reported through the research for the Tripartite Relationship Theory, voice hearers experience their troublesome voices as largely bullying. Getting to grips with first understanding this bullying quality and then working with it is the task of voice hearers who can successfully transform their relationships with voices and then themselves. Where does it start? It is a reciprocal process rather like unknotting a large ball of string. Pulling on one part causes tension elsewhere. But with patience and exploring aspects of the tripartite relationship that may be compromised, the keys to calming the bully and finding an allie instead may be achieved.

We close by offering some reflections from RL specifically related to her voice hearing experiences during the process of writing this book (see Box 10.1), and then by quoting some of the experiences from people, who you may remember from Chapter 3 and who kindly shared their voice hearing experiences during the development of the Tripartite Relationship Theory. We hope this illustrates a narrative in which, although voices can be incredibly distressing, through an array of approaches these experiences can improve.

Box 10.1   RLs' reflections regarding voice hearing during the writing of this book

RL's reflections

The experience of writing this book has been an incredible journey and through it, I have got to know many of my voices a little better and they in turn have both helped and held up the writing process. Listening to them when they are helpful is easy and listening to them when I experience them as contradictory is necessary or it becomes difficult to proceed.

Many voice hearers will recognise the difficulty of trying to undertake a task whilst being regularly interrupted. The act of writing has provoked different voices in various ways, and I have experienced voices being very interested or anxious, derisory or angry. Some voices have also been very directly supportive. For example, George was very encouraging when I was completing the voice profile in Chapter 6. Grande was very helpful in reminding me of his first experience of mark-making with me, described in Chapter 8. These occasions have been joyous and collaborative. I believe these various responses parallel most voice hearers experience of trying to make sense of their voices as well as trying to get on with everyday tasks that require thinking and language.

As the title of Chapter 5 states: "We're in it together" and I was ever conscious of this parallel when I was grappling with words to describe what I wanted to say to voice hearers and their supporters whilst hearing voices reacting to what I was writing. The only way was to work with it and listen at times in case I was missing anything vital. This became very critical for several months whilst attempting to articulate aspects of voice hearing that relate to shame, and indeed my intention was that this theme would occupy most of a chapter. My strong belief is that shame plays a critical role in the voice hearing experience, and possibly for some people, an integral part of why voices emerged in the first place. I state this carefully as this is an untested hypothesis but I can see how very early shame has played a part in the original events that contributed to my voice hearing experience. Whilst trying to articulate the complexity of this emotion and its potential impact on the experience for some voice hearers, several of my voices were extremely interruptive and it became very difficult to write and think clearly about it. I understand this now as primarily their anxiety and feelings of vulnerability. In fact, they are reacting right now. Yet again, the process of writing this book has reminded me of the difficulty every voice hearer faces in living with distressing voices. Sometimes, a break-through in your voice hearing experience includes going near to the edge of your tolerance in order to discover something critical about the relationship between yourself and a voice. Part of the solution to this discomfort is to not always go through it alone. Instead, try to build helpful relationships so that it's possible to explore these difficulties without being destabilised. Building a healthy relationship is an art and involves daring but the ease in your internal world can be mirrored by your voices, as my hunch is that healthy relating is what they ultimately strive for too.

No matter where one might be in terms of their voice hearing experience, whether hearing voices for the first time or for several years, the experience can be distressing, which was captured by Alan during his discussion about his voices: "he's my tormentor"; "he's been telling me to kill myself and do everybody a favour"; "he doesn't turn off, it just doesn't affect him, he just keeps going on"; "there's nothing anybody can do to help" (Alan). A fundamentally important change one can make to address this and to reduce this level of difficulty is to recognise the importance of, and take action towards, regaining one's own agency. Clare recognised this when she shared her experiences and reported: "I've got to take control of myself, I have to empower myself" (Clare). We believe this importantly contributes towards changing these difficult experiences and which can involve a variety of different approaches. This can include taking part in talking therapy and receiving

mental health practitioner support, as reported by Noel: "[talking] helped a lot"...
"I can't thank [therapist and mental health practitioner] enough, they've both really
helped me" (Noel). Alternatively, Diane expressed her self-agency and found sup-
port through sharing her experiences with her peers: "I went to the Hearing Voices
Group and admitted that I was hearing voices, the shame scale came a lot down";
"I think it was the shame of keeping secrets" (Diane).

Perhaps Frank found the most interesting alternative way to regain his sense of
control over his voice hearing experience:

> "I came to see them as different parts of myself, like split off parts of my person-
> ality, basically whenever I've had tragedy in my life, my personality has split off
> at that point and it's become a voice"; "I had to find out who they actually were,
> because until you find out who they are, you don't know how to deal with them.
> So I started questioning them and asking them things in meditation and mindful-
> ness, I spent quite a lot of time just having them shout and yell and scream at me
> before they actually gave me an answer, but eventually they told me who they
> were and I've been able to deal with them a lot better since then"; "I created
> this mind...this garden in my mind for them so that they're all comfortable....
> now when I want to talk to my voices, I go to the garden myself and I talk to
> my voices in the garden and I found that I have a much better conversation with
> them there, because they're not out and seeing everything and being scared and
> they're in this nice relaxing place with a nice pool and trees and tree house and
> all sorts of nice things there, nice little stream."
>
> (Frank)

Preparing for and writing for this book has led us to think about many things. The
gaps in knowledge and research have helped us clarify where we wish to focus
our attention next. Of particular interest to us concerns the anxiety and shame that
voice hearers experience, and about which supporters can struggle, and we believe
it is important to understand what these emotions relate to so we can further support voice hearers and practitioners through our future work. We hope you have
enjoyed reading our work and have found it helpful. We look forward to contributing to future debates regarding the complex but fascinating phenomenon of voice
hearing.

Appendix

Synthesising the experiences of people distressed by voice hearing and practitioners

To complete the development of a theoretical explanation of voice hearing experiences within a mental healthcare context, the two sets of information that were analysed and discussed in Chapters 3 and 4 were brought together as a whole. This involved three stages. First, one of us (Rob Allison) revisited all the coding from the interviews with people who heard voices and from the focus groups of practitioners. Upon reviewing these collectively, it became clear that the coding collectively encapsulated voice hearers' and practitioners' experiences about similar issues but from different perspectives. These were complimentary of one another. So, for example, both in the individual interviews with voice hearers and in the focus group discussions with practitioners, participants shared how difficult they found talking about voices. Second, these two sets of coding were then compared with one another to develop alignment regarding complimentary experiences between the voice hearer and practitioner sets of coding. This involved using the theoretical coding from the voice hearer interviews as a starting point. Then, listed on either side of this, the voice hearer focused coding and the voice hearer initial coding was placed on the left-hand side and the practitioner focused coding and the practitioner initial coding was placed on the right-hand side. An example of this can be seen in Table A.1. In this table, two of the theoretical codes developed from the interviews with voice hearers (Making sense of voices; Biomedical treatment: limited involvement or fearing enforcement) are listed in the middle column and the focused and initial codes related to this for the voice hearers are listed in the columns to the left of this. Following the comparison of codes during the first stage, a decision was made in this second stage to tentatively align the practitioner coding in relation to the voice hearer coding. In the case of the two examples tabulated below, listed to the right of the voice hearer theoretical codes are the focused and initial codes of the practitioners that relate to "Making sense of voices" and "Biomedical treatment".

Table A.1 Example of synthesis of coding

VH initial code	VH focused code	VH theoretical code	Practitioner focused code	Practitioner initial code
Feeling physical presence of voices	Making sense of voices	**Making sense of voices**	Privileging practitioners' interpretations	Constructing voice hearing within a professional framework
Identifying voices as part of self				
Linking voices with trauma				Practitioner knows best
Living with voices				Taking a team approach
Framing experiences according to professional interpretation	Practitioners not talking about voices			
Being persuaded to take medication	Dominating influence of medication	**Biomedical treatment: limited involvement or fearing enforcement**	Dominating medication treatment for voice hearing	Lack of treatment choice
Benefiting from medication				Medicalising and medicating
Coming off medication without support				Medication traps people in MH services
Medication not helping voices				Voice hearing is stigmatised more than other MH problems
Feeling worse from medication				
Medication suppressing emotions				
Wanting to reduce or stop medication				

Following an iterative process of comparing the codes on either side of the middle column (the voice hearer theoretical coding), in which code names and selected quotations were re-read, the alignment of the codes was ordered so that the voice hearer theoretical coding encapsulated both the voice hearers' and the practitioners' complimentary experiences.

Through reviewing the coding in this way, it became clear that not only did the voice hearer and practitioner participants share similar experiences, but they were often misaligned with one another with a different agenda and, unfortunately, typically skirted around core issues underlying voice hearing. For example, practitioners reported they administered medication sometimes because they feared the consequences of failing to administer it and/or they wanted to stop the voice hearing. Voice hearers, on the other hand, reported they took medication because they feared the consequences of failing to accept it but also their voices felt threatened by practitioners' attempts to get rid of them.

The final stage of synthesising the analyses involved crafting and revising from the coding a written theoretical explanation of voice hearing. This led to the merging of some of the codes to elevate the coding beyond the previous two sets of analyses. For example, you may remember, the voice hearer coding included a theoretical code called "Practitioners' actions", which included two sub-themes (Practitioners failing to connect and understand and Practitioners not talking about voices). These two sub-themes were reallocated to other theoretical codes (Practitioners failing to connect and understand merged with "Relating"; Practitioners not talking about voices merged with "Making sense of voices"), thus removing the "Practitioners' actions" theoretical code. It also was clear that the theoretical code "Personal bully" only applied to voice hearers and not practitioners.

This final revision not only strengthened the synthesis of the voice hearers' and practitioners' experiences, but it also encapsulated a broader tripartite relationship between voice hearer, their voice(s), and practitioner. As such, it also became evident that the name of the more abstract theoretical coding had to be re-named to represent the shift from an individual-centric explanation of voice hearing to the 'whole' experience conceptualised within this broader relational and clinical context. The final theoretical coding is presented below in Table A.2.

Table A.2 Completion of theoretical coding

Theoretical codes before synthesis (6)	Themes (and sub-themes) after synthesis (5)
Relating	**1 Interpersonal dynamic** (Extent of collaboration; Acknowledging or avoiding voices)
Making sense of voices	**2 Who's making sense** (Dominant narratives; Collective search for meaning)
Biomedical treatment: limited involvement or fearing enforcement	**3 Medication: helping or hindering** (Agreement on its purpose; Control over treatment decisions; Lack of alternative)
Agency	**4 Level of agency** (Constrained by coercion; Varying ability to influence change)
Personal bully *Practitioners' actions*	**5 Personal bully** *(merged with "Interpersonal dynamic" and "Who's making sense")*

References

Aléx, L., & Hammarström, A. (2008). Shift in power during an interview situation: Methodological reflections inspired by Foucault and Bourdieu. *Nursing Inquiry*, 15(2), 169–176.

Allison, R. (2022). A tripartite relationship theory of voice hearing: A grounded theory study. *Psychosis*, 16(1), 65–77.

Allison, R., & Flemming, K. (2019). Mental health patients' experiences of softer coercion and its effects on their interactions with practitioners: A qualitative evidence synthesis. *Journal of Advanced Nursing*.

Andreasen, N. (1985). *The broken brain*. Harper Collins.

Association, B. M. (2016). *Health in all policies: Health, austerity and welfare reform. A briefing from the board of science*. British Medical Association.

Beavan, V. (2013). Myriad voices, myriad meanings: Review of the research into the subjective experience of hearing voices. In J. Geekie, P. Randal, D. Lampshire, & J. Read, *Experiencing psychosis* (pp. 146–154). Routledge.

Beavan, V., Read, J., & Cartwright, C. (2011). The prevalence of voice-hearers in the general population: A literature review. *Journal of Mental Health*, 20(3), 281–292.

Bentall, R. P. (2009). *Doctoring the mind: Why psychiatric treatments fail*. Penguin UK.

Bentall, R., & Varese, F. (2013). Psychotic hallucinations. In F. Macpherson, & D. Platchias, *Hallucinations: Philosophy and psychology* (p. Ch.4). The MIT Press.

Birchwood, M., & Chadwick, P. (1997). The omnipotence of voices: Testing the validity of a cognitive model. *Psychological Medicine*, 27(6), 1345–1353.

Birks, M., & Mills, J. (2015). *Grounded theory: A practical guide*. Sage.

Bland, R. C., & Parker, J. H. (1978). Prognosis in schizophrenia: Prognostic predictors and outcome. *Archives of General Psychiatry*, 35(1), 72–77.

Bless, J. J., Larøi, F., Laloyaux, J., Kompus, K., Kråkvik, B., Vedul-Kjelsås, E., ... Hugdahl, K. (2018). Do adverse life events at first onset of auditory verbal hallucinations influence subsequent voice characteristics? Results from an epidemiological study. *Psychiatry Research*, 261, 232–236.

Bogen-Johnston, L., Devisser, R., Strauss, C., & Hayward, M. (2020). A qualitative study exploring how Practitioners within Early Intervention in Psychosis Services engage with Service Users' experiences of voice hearing? *Journal of Psychiatric and Mental Health Nursing*, 27(5), 607–615.

Brewin, C. R., Phillips, K., Morton, J., Mason, A. J., Saunders, R., & Longden, E. (2022). Multiplicity in the experience of voice-hearing: A phenomenological inquiry. *Journal of Psychiatric Research*, 156, 564–569.

Care, T. C. (2015). *Improving acute inpatient psychiatric care for adults in England. Interim report*. London.

Ceraso, A., Lin, J. J., Schneider-Thoma, J., Siafis, S., Tardy, M., Komossa, K., ... Leucht, S. (2020). *Maintenance treatment with antipsychotic drugs for schizophrenia*. The Cochrane Database of Systematic Reviews.

Chadwick, P., & Birchwood, M. (1994). The omnipotence of voices: A cognitive approach to auditory hallucinations. *The British Journal of Psychiatry*, 164, 190–201.

Charmaz, K. (2014). *Constructing grounded theory*. Sage.

Choong, C., Hunter, M., & Woodruff, P. (2007). Auditory hallucinations in those populations that do not suffer from schizophrenia. *Current Psychiatry Reports*, 9(3), 206–212.

Coffey, M. & Hewitt, J. (2008). 'You don't talk about the voices': Voice hearers and community mental health nurses talk about responding to voice hearing experiences. *Journal of Clinical Nursing*, 17, 1591–1600.

Coleman, R., & Smith, M. (1997). *Working with voices: Victim to victor*. Handsell.

Cooke, A., Smythe, W., & Anscombe, P. (2019). Conflict, compromise and collusion: Dilemmas for psychosocially-oriented practitioners in the mental health system. *Psychosis*, 11(3), 199–211.

Corstens, D., Longden, E., & May, R. (2012). Talking with voices: Exploring what is expressed by the voices people hear. *Psychology and Psychotherapy: Theory, Research and Practice*, 76(4), 369–383.

Corstens, D., Longden, E., McCarthy-Jones, S., Waddingham, R., & Thomas, N. (2014). Emerging perspectives from the hearing voices movement: Implications for research and practice. *Schizophrenia Bulletin*, 40(Suppl_4), S285–S294.

CQC. (2011). *Monitoring the Mental Health Act in 2010/11*. Care Quality Commission.

CQC. (2013). *Monitoring the Mental Health Act in 2011/12*. Care Quality Commission.

CQC. (2014). *Monitoring the Mental Health Act in 2012/13*. Care Quality Commission.

CQC. (2015). *Monitoring the Mental Health Act in 2013/14*. Care Quality Commission.

CQC. (2016). *Monitoring the Mental Health Act in 2014/15*. Care Quality Commission.

CQC. (2017). *Monitoring the Mental Health Act in 2015/16*. Care Quality Commission.

Craig, T. K., Rus-Calafell, M., Ward, T., Leff, J. P., Huckvale, M., Howarth, E., ... Garety, P. A. (2018). AVATAR therapy for auditory verbal hallucinations in people with psychosis: A single-blind, randomised controlled trial. *The Lancet Psychiatry*, 5(1), 31–40.

Crisp, N., Smith, G., & Nicholson, K. (2016). *Old problems. New solutions: Improving acute psychiatric care for adults in England (The commission on acute adult psychiatric care)*. The Royal College of Psychiatrists.

Cummins, I. (2018). The impact of austerity on mental health service provision: A UK perspective. *International Journal of Environmental Research and Public Health*, 15, 1145.

Daalman, K., Diederen, K. M., Derks, E. M., van Lutterveld, R., Kahn, R. S., & Sommer, I. E. (2012). Childhood trauma and auditory verbal hallucinations. *Psychological Medicine*, 42(12), 2475–2484.

Davies, J. (2021). *Sedated: How modern capitalism created our mental health crisis. Atlantic Books*. Atlantic Books Ltd.

Davies, J., Pace, B. A., & Devenot, N. (2023). Beyond the psychedelic hype: Exploring the persistence of the neoliberal paradigm. *Journal of Psychedelic Studies*, 7(S1), 9–21.

Delespaul, P., deVries, M., & van Os, J. (2002). Determinants of occurrence and recovery from hallucinations in daily life. *Social Psychiatry and Psychiatric Epidemiology*, 37, 97–104.

Department of Health and Social Care (2018). *Independent Review of the Mental Health Act 1983. Modernising the Mental Health Act. Increasing choice, reducing compulsion.* Final report of the Independent Review of the Mental Health Act 1983. https://www.gov.uk/government/publications/modernising-the-mental-health-act-final-report-from-the-independent-review

Dillon, J. (2012). Recovery from "psychosis". In J. Geekie, P. Randal, D. Lampshire, & J. Read, *Experiencing psychosis: Personal and professional perspectives* (pp. 17–22). Routledge.

Dillon, J., & Hornstein, G. A. (2013). Hearing voices peer support groups: A powerful alternative for people in distress. *Psychosis, 5,* 286–295.

Driessen, E., Hollon, S. D., Bockting, C. L., Cuijpers, P., & Turner, E. H. (2015). Does publication bias inflate the apparent efficacy of psychological treatment for major depressive disorder? A systematic review and meta-analysis of US National Institutes of Health-funded trials. *PLoS One, 10,* e0137864.

Esposito, L., & Perez, F. M. (2014). Neoliberalism and the commodification of mental health. *Humanity & Society, 38*(4), 414–442.

Fiorillo, A., & Gorwood, P. (2020). The consequences of the COVID-19 pandemic on mental health and implications for clinical practice. *European Psychiatry, 63*(1), e32.

Fleming, M. P., & Martin, C. R. (2011). Genes and schizophrenia: A pseudoscientific disenfranchisement of the individual. *Journal of Psychiatric and Mental Health Nursing, 18*(6), 469–478.

Foley, T. (2013). *Bridging the gap: The financial case for a reasonable rebalancing of health and care resources.* London.

Garety, P. A., Fowler, D. G., Freeman, D., Bebbington, P., Dunn, G., & Kuipers, E. (2008). Cognitive-behavioural therapy and family intervention for relapse prevention and symptom reduction in psychosis: Randomised controlled trial. *The British Journal of Psychiatry, 192*(6), 412–423.

Gilburt, H. (2015). *Mental health under pressure.* The King's Fund.

Glover-Thomas, N. (2013). The Health and Social Care Act 2012: The emergence of equal treatment for mental health care or another false dawn? *Medical Law International, 13*(4), 279–297.

Goldacre, B. (2010). *Bad science: Quacks, hacks, and big pharma flacks.* McClelland & Stewart.

Goldacre, B. (2014). *Bad pharma: How drug companies mislead doctors and harm patients.* Macmillan.

Hardy, A., Keen, N., van den Berg, D., Varese, F., Longden, E., Ward, T., & Brand, R. M. (2023). Trauma therapies for psychosis: A state-of-the-art review. *Psychology and Psychotherapy: Theory, Research and Practice, 97*(1), 74–90.

Harris, B. A. & Panozzo, G. (2019). Therapeutic alliance, relationship building, and communication strategies-for the schizophrenia population: an integrative review. *Archives of Psychiatric Nursing, 33,* 104–111.

Harrison, G., Hopper, K. I., Craig, T., Laska, E., Siegel, C., Wanderling, J. O., … Wiersma, D. (2001). Recovery from psychotic illness: A 15-and 25-year international follow-up study. *The British Journal of Psychiatry, 178*(6), 506–517.

Harrow, M., Jobe, T. H., Faull, R. N., & Yang, J. (2017). A 20-year multi-followup longitudinal study assessing whether antipsychotic medications contribute to work functioning in schizophrenia. *Psychiatry Research, 256,* 267–274.

Hayward, M. (2003). Interpersonal relating and voice hearing: To what extent does relating to the voice reflect social relating? *Psychology and Psychotherapy: Theory, Research and Practice, 76*(4), 369–383.

Hayward, M., Berry, K., McCarthy-Jones, S., Strauss, C., & Thomas, N. (2014). Beyond the omnipotence of voices: Further developing a relational approach to auditory hallucinations. *Psychosis*, 6(3), 242–252.

Heale, R., & Wray, J. (2020). Mental health in the time of COVID-19. *Evidence-Based Nursing*, 23(4), 93–93.

Health, N. C. (2012). *Service user experience in adult mental health: NICE guidance on improving the experience of care for people using adult NHS mental health services.* RCPsych Publications.

Hearn, J. (2012). *Theorizing Power.* Palgrave Macmillan.

Jauhar, S., McKenna, P. J., Radua, J., Fung, E., Salvador, R., & Laws, K. R. (2014). Cognitive–behavioural therapy for the symptoms of schizophrenia: Systematic review and meta-analysis with examination of potential bias. *The British Journal of Psychiatry*, 204(1), 20–29.

Johns, L. C., Kompus, K., Connell, M., Humpston, C., Lincoln, T. M., Longden, E., ... Larøi, F. (2014). Auditory verbal hallucinations in persons with and without a need for care. *Schizophrenia Bulletin*, 40(Suppl_4), S255–264.

Johnson, S., Gilburt, H., Lloyd-Evans, B., Osborn, D. P., Boardman, J., Leese, M., ... Slade, M. (2009). In-patient and residential alternatives to standard acute psychiatric wards in England. *The British Journal of Psychiatry*, 194(5), 456–463.

Johnstone, L. (2009). Controversial issues in trauma and psychosis. *Psychosis*, 1, 185–190.

Johnstone, L., & Boyle, M. (2018). *The power threat meaning framework: Towards the identification of patterns in emotional distress, unusual experiences and troubled or troubling behaviour, as an alternative to functional psychiatric diagnosis.* British Psychological Society.

Kallert, T., Monahan, J., & Mezzich, J. (2007). World Psychiatric Association (WPA) Thematic Conference: Coercive Treatment in Psychiatry: A Comprehensive Review. Meeting abstracts, Dresden, Germany. 6–8 June 2007. *BMC Psychiatry*, 7 (Supplement 1).

Kamp, K. S., O'Connor, M., Spindler, H., & Moskowitz, A. (2019). Bereavement hallucinations after the loss of a spouse: Associations with psychopathological measures, personality and coping style. *Death Studies*, 43(4), 260–269.

Karanikolos, M., Heino, P., McKee, M., Stuckler, D., & Legido-Quigley, H. (2016). Effects of the global financial crisis on health in high-income OECD countries: A narrative review. *International Journal of Health Services*, 46(2), 208–240.

Kotov, R., Fochtmann, L. L., Tanenberg-Karant, M., Constantino, E. A., Rubinstein, J., Perlman, G., ... Bromet, E. J. (2017). Declining clinical course of psychotic disorders over the two decades following first hospitalization: Evidence from the Suffolk County Mental Health Project. *American Journal of Psychiatry*, 174(11), 1064–1074.

Kråkvik, B., Larøi, F., Kalhovde, A. M., Hugdahl, K., Kompus, K., Salvesen, Ø., ... Vedul-Kjelsås, E. (2015). Prevalence of auditory verbal hallucinations in a general population: A group comparison study. *Scandinavian Journal of Psychology*, 56(5), 508–515.

Lafferty, R. & Grande (2018). Chaos I. Leeds Arts University, UK.

Lafferty, R., & Allison, R. (2021). Voice dialogue. In I. Parker, J. Schnackenberg, & M. Hopfenbeck, *The practical handbook of hearing voices: Therapeutic and creative approaches* (pp. 194–202). PCCS Books.

Lardinois, M., Lataster, T., Mengelers, R., Van Os, J., & Myin-Germeys, I. (2011). Childhood trauma and increased stress sensitivity in psychosis. *Acta Psychiatrica Scandinavica*, 123(1), 28–35.

Larkin, W., & Read, J. (2008). Childhood trauma and psychosis: Evidence, pathways, and implications. *Journal of Postgraduate Medicine*, 54(4), 287–293.

Larøi, F. (2012). How do auditory verbal hallucinations in patients differ from those in non-patients? *Frontiers in Human Neuroscience*, 6, 25.

Larøi, F., Sommer, I. E., Blom, J. D., Fernyhough, C., Ffytche, D. H., Hugdahl, K., ... Waters, F. (2012). The characteristic features of auditory verbal hallucinations in clinical and nonclinical groups: State-of-the-art overview and future directions. *Schizophrenia Bulletin*, 38(4), 724–733.

Lataster, T., van Os, J., Drukker, M., enquet, C., Feron, F., Gunther, N., & Myin-Germeys, I. (2006). Childhood victimisation and developmental expression of non-clinical delusional ideation and hallucinatory experiences: Victimisation and non-clinical psychotic experiences. *Social Psychiatry and Psychiatric Epidemiology*, 41, 423–428.

Lawrence, C., Jones, J., & Cooper, M. (2010). Hearing voices in a non-psychiatric population. *Behavioural and Cognitive Psychotherapy*, 38(3), 363–373.

Linscott, R. J., & Van Os, J. (2013). An updated and conservative systematic review and meta-analysis of epidemiological evidence on psychotic experiences in children and adults: On the pathway from proneness to persistence to dimensional expression across mental disorders. *Psychological Medicine*, 43(6), 1133–1149.

Luhrmann, T. M., Alderson-Day, B., Bell, V., Bless, J. J., Corlett, P., Hugdahl, K., ... Waters, F. (2019). Beyond trauma: A multiple pathways approach to auditory hallucinations in clinical and nonclinical populations. *Schizophrenia Bulletin*, 45(Supplement_1), S24–S31.

Mahase, E. (2020). *Workforce crisis has left mental health staff at "breaking point" as demand rises.* British Medical Journal Publishing Group.

Mawson, A., Berry, K., Murray, C., & Hayward, M. (2011). Voice hearing within the context of hearers' social worlds: An interpretative phenomenological analysis. *Psychology and Psychotherapy: Theory, Research and Practice*, 84, 256–272.

May, R., & Svanholmer, E. (2019, September). *Self-help guide to talking with voices.* Retrieved from https://openmindedonline.com/wp-content/uploads/2019/09/self-help-guide-to-talking-with-voices-r.-may-and-e.-svanholmer-sep-2019.pdf

McCarthy-Jones, S., & Longden, E. (2013). The voices others cannot hear. *Psychologist*, 26, 570–574.

McCrone, P., Dhanasiri, S., Patel, A., Knapp, M., & Lawton-Smith, S. (2008). *Paying the price: The cost of mental health care in England to 2026.* The King's Fund.

McManus, S., Bebbington, P., Jenkins, R., & Brugha, T. (2016). *Mental health and wellbeing in England: Adult Psychiatric Morbidity Survey 2014.* A survey carried out for NHS Digital by NatCen Social Research and the Department of Health Sciences, Universit.

McMullan, E., Gupta, A., & Collins, S. (2018). Experiences of mental health nursing staff working with voice hearers in an acute setting: An interpretive phenomenological approach. *Journal of Psychiatric and Mental Health Nursing*, 25, 157–166.

Mills, J., Bonner, A., & Francis, K. (2006). The development of constructivist grounded theory. *International Journal of Qualitative Methods*, 5, 25–35.

Moilanen, J., Haapea, M., Miettunen, J., Jääskeläinen, E., Veijola, J., Isohanni, M., & Koponen, H. (2013). Characteristics of subjects with schizophrenia spectrum disorder with and without antipsychotic medication–A 10-year follow-up of the Northern Finland 1966 British Cohort Study. *European Psychiatry*, 28(1), 53–58.

Moncrieff, J. (2008). *The myth of the chemical cure: A critique of psychiatric drug.* MacMillan.

Morgan, C., Fearon, P., Lappin, J., Heslin, M., Donoghue, K., Lomas, B., ... Dazzan, P. (2017). Ethnicity and long-term course and outcome of psychotic disorders in a UK sample: The ÆSOP-10 study. *The British Journal of Psychiatry*, 211(2), 88–94.

Navarro, V. (2007). Neoliberalism as a class ideology; or, the political causes of the growth of inequalities. *International Journal of Health Services*, 37(1), 47–62.

Nettleton, S. (2021). *The sociology of health and illness*. Polity Press.

NHS (2019). *The NHS long term plan*. https://www.longtermplan.nhs.uk/

NICE. (2014). *Psychosis and schizophrenia in adults: Treatment and management*. NICE.

NICE. (2015). *Violence and aggression: Short-term management in mental health, health and community settings*. NICE.

NMC. (2015). *The code: Professional standards of practice and behaviour for nurses and midwives*. Nursing and Midwifery Council.

Pansardi, P. (2012). Power to and power over: Two distinct concepts of power? *Journal of Political Power*, 5(1), 73–89.

Peplau, H. (1991). *Interpersonal relations in nursing: A conceptual frame of reference for psychodynamic nursing*. Springer Publishing Company.

Peplau, H. (1992). Interpersonal relations: A theoretical framework for application in nursing practice. *Nursing Science Quarterly*, 5, 13–18.

Pierre, J. (2010). Hallucinations in nonpsychotic disorders: Toward a differential diagnosis of "hearing voices". *Harvard Review of Psychiatry*, 18, 22–35.

Pontillo, M., De Crescenzo, F., Vicari, S., Pucciarini, M. L., Averna, R., Santonastaso, O., & Armando, M. (2016). Cognitive behavioural therapy for auditory hallucinations in schizophrenia: A review. *World Journal of Psychiatry*, 6(3), 372.

Rácz, J., Kaló, Z., Kassai, S., Kiss, M., & Pintér, J. N. (2017). The experience of voice hearing and the role of self-help group: An interpretative phenomenological analysis. *International Journal of Social Psychiatry*, 63(4), 307–313.

RCP. (2014). *Good psychiatric practice: Code of ethics*. Royal College of Psychiatrist.

Read, J., & Bentall, R. (2012). Negative childhood experiences and mental health: Theoretical, clinical and primary prevention implications. *The British Journal of Psychiatry*, 200(2), 89–91.

Romme, M., & Escher, S. (1993). *Accepting voices*. MIND.

Romme, M., & Escher, S. (2000). *Making sense of voices: The mental health professional's guide to working with voice-hearers*. Mind Publications.

Romme, M., Escher, S., Dillon, J., Corstens, D., & Morris, M. (2009). *Living with voices: 50 stories of recovery*. PCCS Books.

Saab, M. M., Murphy, M., Meehan, E., Dillon, C. B., O'Connell, S., Hegarty, J., Heffernan, S., Greaney, S., Kilty, C., Goodwin, J., & Hartigan, I. (2022). Suicide and self-harm risk assessment: A systematic review of prospective research. *Archives of Suicide Research*, 26(4), 1645–1665.

Sharma, T., Guski, L. S., Freund, N., & Gøtzsche, P. C. (2016). Suicidality and aggression during antidepressant treatment: Systematic review and meta-analyses based on clinical study reports. *BMJ*, 352, i65.

Shorter, E. (1998). *History of psychiatry: From the era of the asylum to the age of prozac*. John Wiley & Sons.

Simpson, A., Allison, R., & Lambley, R. (2017). The acute care setting. In M. Chambers, *Psychiatric and mental health nursing: The craft of caring*, 3rd ed. (Ch. 53, pp. 587–594). Routledge.

Sommer, I. E., Daalman, K., Rietkerk, T., Diederen, K. M., Bakker, S., Wijkstra, J., ... Boks, M. P. (2010). Healthy individuals with auditory verbal hallucinations; who are they? Psychiatric assessments of a selected sample of 103 subjects. *Schizophrenia Bulletin*, 36(3), 633–641.

Stone, H., & Stone, S. (1989). *Embracing our selves: The voice dialogue manual*. New World Library.

Thomas, N., Hayward, M., Peters, E., Van Der Gaag, M., Bentall, R. P., Jenner, J., ... McCarthy-Jones, S. (2014). Psychological therapies for auditory hallucinations (voices): current status and key directions for future research. *Schizophrenia Bulletin*, 40(Suppl_4), S202–S212.

Thornicroft, G. (2000). National service framework for mental health. *Psychiatric Bulletin*, 24, 203–206.

Varese, F., Smeets, F., Drukker, M., Lieverse, R., Lataster, T., Viechtbauer, W., ... Bentall, R. P. (2012). Childhood adversities increase the risk of psychosis: A meta-analysis of patient-control, prospective-and cross-sectional cohort studies. *Schizophrenia Bulletin*, 38(4), 661–671.

Waters, F. (2010). Auditory hallucinations in psychiatric illness. *Psychiatric Times*, 27(3), 54.

Waters, F., & Fernyhough, C. (2017). Hallucinations: A systematic review of points of similarity and difference across diagnostic classes. *Schizophrenia Bulletin*, 43, 32–43.

Wilkinson, S., & Krueger, J. (2022). The phenomenology of voice-hearing and two concepts of voice. In A. Woods, B. Alderson-Day, & C. Fernyhough, *Voices in psychosis: Interdisciplinary perspectives* (pp. 127–133). Oxford University Press.

Wils, R. S., Gotfredsen, D. R., Hjorthøj, C., Austin, S. F., Albert, N., Secher, R. G., ... Nordentoft, M. (2017). Antipsychotic medication and remission of psychotic symptoms 10 years after a first-episode psychosis. *Schizophrenia Research*, 182, 42–48.

Wood, L., & Alsawy, S. (2016). Patient experiences of psychiatric inpatient care: A systematic review of qualitative evidence. *Journal of Psychiatric Intensive Care*, 12(1), 35–43.

Woods, A. (2013). The voice-hearer. *Journal of Mental Health*, 22(3), 263–270.

Woods, A., Jones, N., Alderson-Day, B., Callard, F., & Fernyhough, C. (2015). Experiences of hearing voices: Analysis of a novel phenomenological survey. *The Lancet Psychiatry*, 2, 323–331.

Index

Note: **Bold** page numbers refer to tables and *italic* page numbers refer to figures.

For Product Safety Concerns and Information please contact our EU
representative GPSR@taylorandfrancis.com
Taylor & Francis Verlag GmbH, Kaufingerstraße 24, 80331 München, Germany

www.ingramcontent.com/pod-product-compliance
Lightning Source LLC
Chambersburg PA
CBHW052009270326
41929CB00015B/2854

9 781032 619842